Praise for
Celiac Disease: A Hidden Epidemic

"A must-read for those with celiac disease and anyone with suspect symptoms (gastrointestinal complaints, anemia, fatigue, headaches, joint pain, etc.). . . . If you buy just one medical book about celiac disease, make it this one."
—*Living Without*

"The book the celiac world has needed all along."
—Gluten Intolerance Group

"The definitive resource for every celiac, those yet to be diagnosed, and their families. Comprehensive and concise, yet easy to understand. This is a must-have book."
—Elaine Monarch, Celiac Disease Foundation

"Easy to read. . . . Full of common sense and suggestions that go to the heart of celiac concerns."
—*Gluten-Free Living*

"An exceptionally complete yet easy to read guide to celiac disease and strategies for living with it successfully. . . . Highly recommended."
—ChildrenWithDiabetes.com

"Useful, in-depth information for sufferers. . . . This book is important for consumer health libraries and consumer health collections in public libraries."
—*Library Journal*

"As director of the Celiac Disease Center at Columbia University, Green's a top expert in one of the most under-diagnosed diseases in America."
—*New York Post*

CELIAC DISEASE

(UPDATED 4TH EDITION)

CELIAC DISEASE

A HIDDEN EPIDEMIC

UPDATED 4TH EDITION

Peter H. R. Green, M.D.,
and Rory Jones, M.S.

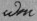
WILLIAM MORROW
An Imprint of HarperCollins*Publishers*

This book contains advice and information relating to health care. It is not intended to replace medical advice and should be used to supplement rather than replace regular care by your doctor. It is recommended that you seek your physician's advice before embarking on any medical program or treatment. All efforts have been made to assure the accuracy of the information contained in this book as of the date of publication. The publisher and the author disclaim liability for any medical outcomes that may occur as a result of applying the methods suggested in this book.

The Library of Congress has cataloged the previous edition as follows:

Green, Peter H. R.
    Celiac disease : a hidden epidemic / Peter H. R. Green and Rory Jones.
—1st ed.
        p. cm.
    ISBN-10: 0-06-076693-X
        1. Celiac disease.   2. Intestines—diseases.

RC862.C44 G74 2006
616.3/99 22
                                                                2006295906

ISBN 978-0-06-303485-3 (pbk.)

23 24 25 26 27 LBC 6 5 4 3 2

HEALTH QUESTIONNAIRE

SECTION I: SYMPTOMS
Check each of the symptoms that you have experienced at least once a week during the past three months:

___ Bloating
___ Gas and/or stomach cramping
___ Diarrhea or runny stools
___ Constipation
___ Joint pain
___ Numbness or tingling in your extremities
___ Itchy skin lesions
___ Constant unexplained fatigue
___ Frequent headaches or migraines

SECTION II: DIAGNOSES
Check if you have had or been diagnosed with any of the following:

___ Irritable bowel syndrome
___ Eczema or unexplained contact dermatitis
___ Fibromyalgia
___ Chronic fatigue syndrome
___ Nervous stomach (non-ulcer dyspepsia)

SECTION III: ASSOCIATED ILLNESSES
Check if you have any of the following:

___ Lactose intolerance
___ Osteopenia and/or osteoporosis
___ Autoimmune disorders
___ Thyroid disease (hypo/hyper)

___ Diabetes mellitus (type 1)
___ Sjögren's syndrome
___ Chronic liver disease
___ An immediate family member with an autoimmune condition
___ Peripheral neuropathy
___ Non-Hodgkin's lymphoma
___ Small intestinal cancer
___ Psychiatric disorders or depression
___ Anemia (iron deficiency)
___ Infertility

SCORING

If you have checked one or more lines in *either* Section I or II and have *any* of the illnesses in Section III (especially males or women under forty-five with osteopenia and/or osteoporosis), you should consider testing for celiac disease. If you have checks in all three sections, you and your doctor(s) should definitely explore a diagnosis of celiac disease.

All of the symptoms in Section I, all of the diagnoses in Section II, and all of the associated illnesses in Section III are intimately related to celiac disease. One in every 100 people in the United States is affected by celiac disease—and about 50 percent of them are undiagnosed!

CONTENTS

ACKNOWLEDGMENTS

This book evolved from the combination of two sometimes diverse perspectives: that of the doctor and the patient. It incorporates an understanding of both the science and the experience of an illness—and the collective knowledge we both have acquired in the process. This revised fourth edition reflects the current developments in a rapidly changing field.

We would like to thank everyone we have worked and collaborated with over the past number of years, but some deserve a special mention.

I appreciate the frequent interactions with my colleagues in the Celiac Disease Center at Columbia University, especially Amy DeFelice, Ben Lebwohl, Suneeta Krishnareddy, Suzanne Lewis, Anne Lee, Jessica Lebovits, Cynthia Beckman, Govind Bhagat, Ed Ciaccio, and Randi Wolf.

—*Peter Green, M.D.*

There are many people who educated me about celiac disease and dermatitis herpetiformis—as well as how to live well with a chronic illness. I am particularly indebted to the many medical professionals, patients, students, and friends who shared their stories that shaped the narratives about living with celiac disease that resonate throughout this book.

As always, my family deserve the deepest thanks for their endless patience and humor, without which nothing would be possible.

—*Rory Jones*

We both want to express special thanks to:

Jennifer Civiletto, our editor, who graciously and tirelessly supplied encouragement and professional guidance; Faith Hamlin, our agent, who championed the book even before she knew that some of her best friends had celiac disease; and Cathy Hemming, whose vision made it possible.

Finally, we want to thank the many patients who so generously gave us their time and shared their insights. This book is for you and the many people living with celiac disease and those making the long journey to diagnosis.

The Celiac Disease Center at Columbia University

The Celiac Disease Center at Columbia University is one of the few leading centers in the United States that provides comprehensive medical care, including nutritional counseling, for adult and pediatric patients with celiac disease. Its mission is to redefine the future of celiac disease and treatment through continuing advances in research, patient care, and physician and public education. The Center is diagnosing and treating more than two thousand patients annually from around the world. In its nineteen years of operation, the Center owes much to the generous individuals who have assisted us in fulfilling its goals.

A NOTE FROM THE AUTHORS

All of the information in this book is based on current knowledge about the causes, manifestations, diagnosis, treatment, and consequences of celiac disease. It is derived from an in-depth analysis of current medical literature, extensive clinical experience, patient and professional interviews, as well as ongoing research into celiac disease and its many complications.

Other medical experts may have differing opinions and interpretations of the medical literature. Wherever pertinent, the authors have attempted to note conflicting points of view on key issues as well as topics that have not as yet been scientifically resolved.

Many of the peer review articles we have consulted may not be readily accessible to all readers. For this reason, we have not included footnotes for all medical facts and figures. Instead, we have listed good basic review articles and books for different subjects in the Appendices.

The personal stories and diagnoses throughout this book are based primarily on the patient population seen at the Celiac Disease Center at Columbia University. The population of the greater New York tristate area is very large and ethnically diverse. In addition, the patients who seek help at a major medical center may present with more severe and complex symptoms. We understand that this may or may not be typical of the celiac profile in any given city or region of the United States. Nevertheless, we feel that the cross section of patients chosen for this book reflects the face of celiac disease in the United States today.

Note: This book is not a self-diagnosis manual. It is intended to generate informed patients who know what questions to ask of their physicians and how to understand the answers.

What's Wrong with Me?

My doctor kept treating my symptoms, but never figured out why my stomach was always upset. I started getting migraines and then joint pain and... well, you name it. I was a walking pharmacy and still felt lousy. (Marg, 47)*

My daughter was always tired. It was a joke with her friends—where's Mel—she's asleep. She slept through classes in college... it affected her social life. We even did an overnight sleep study in the hospital—she was sleeping fourteen to sixteen hours a day. (Roni)

My daughter had legs like pick-up sticks and an enormous belly and the pediatrician called it "baby fat" and said she'd grow into it. (Mike, 40)

I think people thought I was a hypochondriac—there was so much wrong with me. (Heather, 43)

In the United States today, millions of patients suffer with symptoms that neither fit a specific diagnosis nor disappear. Young and old take drugs and see numerous specialists for gastrointestinal complaints, anemia, joint pain, itchy skin conditions, constant fatigue, or headaches. Their symptoms are treated, but no underlying cause can be found. One doctor diagnoses fibromyalgia, another chronic fatigue syndrome, a third irritable bowel syndrome. Too much or too little roughage, lactose or

---

* In order to preserve patient confidentiality we have used first names or pseudonyms throughout. Some patients declined to have their ages listed.

fructose intolerance, fried or spicy food explains repeated bouts of reflux, diarrhea, constipation, abdominal pain, and gas. Muscle strain or the "wrong type of mattress" is the excuse for aching joints or tingling extremities that remain asleep when the rest of you wakes up in the morning.

Frustrated, patients seek care from "alternative" nontraditional physicians because a friend or neighbor got help there or the physician appeared on TV. Hundreds of dollars later—after a battery of blood or stool tests that most traditional physicians will not even review once they see the name of the laboratory that performed them—the diagnosis comes down to "leaky" gut or too much of the wrong bacteria. Trials of antibacterial agents, expensive intravenous vitamin infusions, multiple herbal remedies, or low-yeast diets all seem the answer. They provide a temporary respite when well-trained physicians cannot provide an answer.

Six or seven years into this downward physical and mental spiral, an internist suggests that stress may be the answer. In other words, we cannot find anything really wrong with you—perhaps it is "in your head." Many patients live in a perpetual state of indefinable ill health that, after a period of time, they begin to accept as normal. Some of the symptoms seem to "run in the family."

> I've had it (reflux and dyspepsia) for so long that I just think it's a normal part of my life. My mother has it, my brother has it. So, I just assume it's what I'm supposed to have. (Cindy, 45)

For many patients, there is a medical diagnosis for the bundle of symptoms they must endure. Diagnosis and treatment of this condition will not only improve your health, it may save your life.

The Celiac Iceberg

Celiac disease is a multisystem disorder whose primary target of injury is the small intestine. The disease is triggered by gluten, the main storage protein found in certain grains. Gluten damages the small intestine so that it is unable to absorb nutrients properly. As food malabsorption continues and the disease progresses, the manifestations inevitably become more varied and complex.

Celiac disease is the most common—and one of the most underdiagnosed—hereditary autoimmune condition in the United States today. It is as common as hereditary high cholesterol.

Once considered a rare "diarrheal" disease of childhood, celiac disease is now recognized predominantly as a disease of adults—and the majority of people are either asymptomatic or consult doctors for a variety of other complaints.

While the disease is considered common in Europe, South America, Canada, and Australia—a recent study of schoolchildren in Finland showed the incidence to be one per ninety-nine, in parts of England one per one hundred—**only recently have studies shown that celiac disease affects approximately 1 percent of the U.S. population (approximately 1 in every 100 people)—and about 50 percent of them are *undiagnosed*.** Unfortunately, if the disease progresses and is not diagnosed until later in adulthood, patients often develop many other problems from years of inflammation and the malabsorption of minerals, vitamins, and other necessary nutrients.

A delay in diagnosis also increases the chances of developing associated autoimmune diseases. Most adults with celiac disease have bone loss, resulting in osteopenia or osteoporosis. Anemia, malignancies, peripheral neuropathies (numb and/or tingling extremities), dental enamel defects, hyposplenism (underactive spleen), and infertility are also secondary conditions associated with the disease.

Since patients with one autoimmune disease are more likely to have or to develop another, patients with celiac disease are also seen with Sjögren's syndrome, type 1 diabetes, autoimmune thyroid disease, dermatitis herpetiformis (an intensely itchy skin condition), or alopecia areata (a condition that causes hair loss). **Of the 1.25 million people with type 1 diabetes, 8 to 10 percent also have celiac disease.**

Often, people are treated for an autoimmune condition before being diagnosed with celiac disease.

Unfortunately, there is an increased mortality rate for people with celiac disease, exceeding that of the general population, due mainly to malignancies. Current research shows a statistical risk that is 33 times greater for small intestinal adenocarcinoma, 11.6 times greater for esophageal cancer, 9.1 times greater for non-Hodgkin's lymphoma, 5 times greater for melanoma, and 23 times greater for papillary thyroid cancer.

In the United States today, **the diagnosis of celiac disease can take five to seven years**. Patients normally see numerous physicians and specialists for symptoms that are misdiagnosed, do not respond to drug therapy, or are treated without concern for their underlying cause. Young children may suffer for one-third to one-half their lifetime before obtaining a diagnosis.

A majority of people in the United States have a "silent" variety of celiac disease. Without marked gastrointestinal symptoms, many of these patients are diagnosed with celiac disease concurrent with another diagnosis, often a malignancy. This scenario also occurs in adults who received a celiac disease diagnosis as a child and whose parents were told they would "grow out of it."

> I was told by my mom—many, many years ago—that I had celiac disease as a baby. I had severe diarrhea and the doctor put me on a special milk and bananas diet and it went away and that was the end of it. When I was diagnosed with celiac disease two years ago, I said: "I had that as a baby." (Linda, 62)

You do not outgrow celiac disease. You develop symptoms that point in other medical directions and become part of the iceberg that is "below the waterline" and off the medical radar screens. Patients often see doctors for a myriad of other complaints, and their mild or apparently unrelated symptoms are often only recognized retrospectively.

"Why Worry?"

Celiac disease is a significant medical condition. It is far too often masked by or mistaken for a number of more commonly diagnosed conditions. The result is a huge population of patients suffering unnecessarily and at considerable risk for major complications. These patients may also be burdened by depression and complicated professional and family dynamics as a result of their long-term undiagnosed illnesses.

Recent research and educational efforts have markedly increased the number of people who are diagnosed with celiac disease. Our efforts now must also concentrate on quality of life—to ensure that those with celiac disease remain happy and healthy.

Celiac disease is a huge iceberg that is moving, not quite so silently, across many of our lives.

PART I

IS THE FOOD YOU EAT EATING YOU?

FOOD: CAN'T LIVE WITHOUT IT, CAN'T ALWAYS DIGEST IT.

Pepto-Bismol, Pepcid AC, Imodium AD . . . I should own stock in these companies.

—Cindy, 45

1

Normal Digestion

A good many things go around in the dark besides Santa Claus.
—Herbert Hoover, 1935

Gas, burps, stomachaches, and bloating are standard fodder for comedy routines—because of their frequency as much as the discomfort and embarrassment they cause. Digestive disorders are among the most common problems we experience. Recent figures show that almost half the U.S. population experiences heartburn regularly, one in five are lactose intolerant, and colon and rectal cancers are second only to lung cancer as a leading cause of cancer deaths.

In order to understand the impact of a malfunction in the digestive tract and why it leads to all of the symptomatic manifestations of celiac disease, it is necessary to understand how the body normally digests and absorbs food.

Food keeps my body running and it keeps me up at night. (Gary, 49)

The digestive system has been described as the outside world going through us. Designed to supply the body with all of the nutrients and fluids it needs to function, it is essentially a long tube that is open at both ends. Food enters at one end, the nutrients the body can use are absorbed by the lining of the gastrointestinal tract, and nondigested residue is excreted from the other end. The concept is simple, the design and execution quite remarkable.

The Gastrointestinal (GI) Tract

Food enters the GI tract via the mouth; moves through the pharynx, esophagus, stomach, small intestine (the duodenum, jejunum, and ileum), and large intestine (colon); and exits from the anus. The salivary glands, pancreas, liver, and gallbladder are organs that secrete the enzymes and fluids that help digest food. They are connected to the digestive system by ducts.

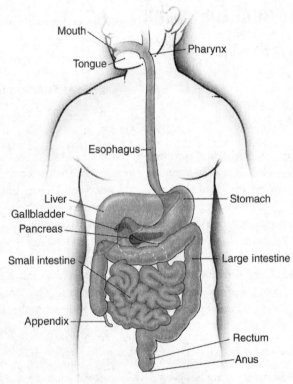

Figure 1. The Digestive Tract
(All illustrations by Thom Graves)

The digestive system, or gut, is intimately related to the following:

- The circulatory system, which transports the nutrients from the intestine to the tissues throughout the body and liver

- The enteric nervous system, which helps control enzyme release and muscular contractions of the gut
- The muscles of the digestive system, which provide motility to help digest and move food through the long tract

If one section of the system malfunctions, it almost necessarily affects another, and there are numerous places for things to go wrong.

Digestion

Digestion is the word commonly used to describe a three-part process:

1. Digestion—the breakdown of food products into ever smaller and smaller components that can be absorbed
2. Absorption—the passage of food products that have been broken down into the intestinal wall
3. Transport—the transfer of food from the intestinal wall to the cells of the body

Digestion requires the following:

- The chemical breakdown of food by enzymes
- The mechanical mixing and propulsion of the products of chemical activity by the intestinal muscle

Digestion actually begins before the food even enters your mouth. When you see, think about, or smell food, the vagus nerve transmits a chemical message from your brain to release saliva in the mouth, increase stomach motility, and release gastric acid in the stomach. We begin to salivate and the stomach "rumbles" at the very anticipation of food.

The Mouth

In the mouth, chewing tears the food apart and grinds it into smaller components. Saliva, a mucous substance, is secreted to lubricate and start to dissolve the food. It contains various enzymes that start the digestion of fats and carbohydrates that are continued farther down the digestive tract. Saliva also acts as a glue to hold the food together as it travels toward the stomach.

We swallow the ball, or *bolus,* of chewed food and saliva, and it is transported down our esophagus. While the skeletal muscles at work in the mouth and throat are voluntary—we consciously move our jaws and swallow—smooth muscles that function involuntarily take over in the esophagus. The gut actually has its own pacemaker. An undulating contraction of muscles called *peristalsis* begins and moves the food into the stomach where the action, quite literally, really starts.

The Stomach

The stomach is a big muscular sac or reservoir that holds the chewed food until it is ready to move on, mixes it with gastric juices, and starts many of the chemical processes of digestion. The muscular movements of the stomach act like a Cuisinart—chopping, blending, and mixing the ball of food to form a soupy puree called *chyme.*

The stomach secretes an enormous amount of *gastric acid,* which functions to both break down the food and convert the stomach into a disinfecting tank, killing bacteria and inactivating toxins in the food we have eaten.

Pepsin, an enzyme secreted by the stomach, starts the digestion of protein.

The stomach also sends messages (in the form of hormones) to the other digestive organs telling them that food has arrived. This stimulates the secretion of pancreatic juices and bile from the liver and gallbladder that will further break down the chyme once it moves into the small intestine. The only substances that are absorbed directly into the bloodstream in the stomach are aspirin and alcohol.

One-Way Street

The *sphincters* that connect the esophagus to the stomach and the stomach to the small intestine are one-way valves. Food is only meant to travel *down* the GI tract—a street sign that is often ignored. Occasionally, chyme refluxes, or backs up, into the esophagus—a condition known as GERD, gastroesophageal reflux disease—and the gastric acid becomes a corrosive agent on the less well-protected lining of the esophagus. (See Chapter 3.)

When the chyme is sufficiently liquefied, muscle/peristaltic contractions gradually push it into the upper part of the small intestine, the *duodenum.* The stomach empties in a slow and controlled way so as not to overwhelm all the mechanisms of digestion in the small intestine.

As the small intestine fills with chyme, it signals the stomach to decrease its activity and slow down the emptying process. This is one reason a large meal "stays with you"; i.e., it lingers in the stomach until the small intestine can process it.

The arrival of chyme in the small intestine triggers the release of specific hormones that stimulate the release of enzymes and fluids into the *lumen,* the center of the tube, to facilitate digestion. The pancreas and the liver supply many of these enzymes and fluids that break down food into components small enough to be absorbed. They are regulated by both the nervous system and gastrointestinal hormones. Their secretions are called for only when needed by the digestive system.

The Pancreas

In addition to its endocrine function (the production of insulin), the pancreas produces enzymes such as *trypsin,* which breaks down proteins; *amylase,* which breaks down starches; and *lipase,* which breaks down fats.

When the pancreas becomes inflamed or diseased (e.g., *pancreatitis*), these enzymes are not secreted and, as a result, carbohydrate, protein, and fat digestion is impaired. (See Pancreatic Insufficiency, Chapter 16.)

The Liver

The liver plays an important role in the metabolism, transport, and storage of nutrients. It assists in the digestion of fats by secreting *bile,* which increases the solubility of fats, enabling them to pass through the intestinal wall into the bloodstream. The bile produced by the liver is stored in the gallbladder until needed; it is delivered to the small intestine on the arrival of fatty foods, which stimulate its release.

The many chemical messengers that stimulate the digestive organs are balanced by a feedback mechanism that turns off production. This delicate balance, or *homeostasis,* controls all digestive functions.

The Small Intestine

The small intestine is the major site for both the digestion (breaking down) and absorption of nutrients. In the average adult, it is approximately twenty-two feet long and consists of three parts:

- The duodenum (the first segment)
- The jejunum (the second segment—together with the duodenum known as the *proximal* intestine)
- The ileum (the third segment or *distal* intestine)

All three segments have similar anatomy, but each has a specific job, digesting and absorbing particular nutrients.

While digestion takes place in the lumen of the small intestine, absorption occurs through the lining or mucosal wall of the intestine, which has a unique structure. The twenty-two feet of small intestine actually possesses a much larger surface area than it would appear.

The lining of the wall of the small intestine, the *mucosa,* consists of folds that markedly increase its surface area. The folds are in turn covered with tiny fingerlike projections, or *villi,* that contain the cells that absorb nutrients. These villi further amplify the surface area.

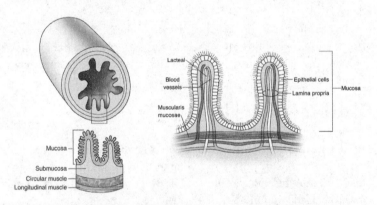

Figures 2 and 3. A Cross Section of the Intestinal Wall

The surface of each villus has a "brushlike" border consisting of *microvilli,* or tiny hairs, that increase the absorptive surface of the small intestine yet again. The brush border also contains enzymes that are necessary for the digestion of specific food components.

If you were to flatten out the intestinal mucosa—all the villi, microvilli, and *crypts* (the small valleys between each villus)—the "small" intestine actually has a surface area about the size of a tennis court that is totally dedicated to absorbing food! This enormous capacity ensures that the intestine can sustain a fair amount of assault and/or damage and still feed the body.

Inflammatory cells normally inhabit the mucosa to protect the small intestine against toxins and bacteria. Since the food supply entering the GI tract is not "sterile" and may contain toxic substances, these white blood cells are the first line of defense. This results in a state of constant controlled inflammation in the mucosa. (See The Burn, Chapter 3.)

The Villi

The villi are the workhorses of the intestine. They are the final intestinal link between your dinner plate and your bloodstream. And this is where celiac disease does its primary damage.

The villi play a crucial role by:

1. Dramatically increasing the surface area of the small intestine to allow the absorption of food
2. Releasing enzymes that continue and complete the breakdown/digestion of food
3. Absorbing the products of digestion and transporting them into the bloodstream for distribution throughout the body
4. Acting as a barrier that blocks bacteria, parasites, and toxins from entering the body

Each villus is an independent, but intimately related part of the assembly line. The villi are made up of epithelial cells that cover a core containing blood and lymph vessels, nerve fibers, and a muscle layer. As illustrated in Figure 2 (page 12), the muscle is both longitudinal (pushing) and circular (mixing). This muscular component consists of smooth muscle that is innately contractile. It is a crucial aspect of digestion, since contractions of the smooth muscle both propel and mix the chyme as it travels down the digestive tract. Without peristalsis, there would be no digestion.

It is important to understand that the final stages of digestion, absorption, and transport of nutrients occur *through*—not between—these tiny, fingerlike projections. When there is inflammation, and a breakdown of the lining of the intestine, the bowel may become "leaky."

This enables whole molecules of food and/or toxins to get *between or through* the epithelial cells, interrupting their protective function. When the lining is intact, larger molecules will not enter the bowel wall and bloodstream.

There are millions of these microscopic villi in each section of the small intestine. Because of its enormous capacity to absorb, parts of it can be damaged with no obvious manifestations or symptoms. This enormous anatomical surplus is designed to compensate for damage to the intestine from any source, infection, poison, or inflammation. But when large sections of the lining are inflamed or destroyed, absorption, enzyme release, transport of nutrients to the body, and the defensive ability of the small intestine are compromised.

Crypts

The small valleys between the villi—crypts—continuously produce and replace the absorptive epithelial cells lining each villus of the GI tract and secrete enzymes into the lumen to aid in digestion. Billions of epithelial cells are replaced every day, but if the villi are inflamed or damaged, new cells are unable to work their way up the villus and the crypts become swollen.

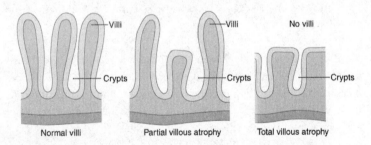

Figure 4. Normal Villi; Partial Villous Atrophy; Total Villous Atrophy

Absorption

Once the food components traveling through the lumen are sufficiently digested (broken down), they are absorbed by different parts of the small intestine.

A disease of or infection in one section of the small intestine is often revealed by the malabsorption of specific nutrients. Iron deficiency and metabolic bone disease (e.g., osteoporosis or osteopenia) occur when disease involves the *proximal intestine*. Fat and sugars also get absorbed in the upper intestine. If they are malabsorbed, and the ileum cannot compensate, they get into the colon and you get diarrhea. (See Chapter 3.) Vitamin B_{12} malabsorption occurs when the ileum is involved in a disease process. This may occur in severe celiac disease or, more commonly, Crohn's disease with ileitis.

Unless there is a disease process at work, the absorption process works efficiently and steadily until every usable nutrient in the chyme is absorbed. Limits are placed only on the absorption of necessary, but potentially toxic minerals such as iron and calcium.

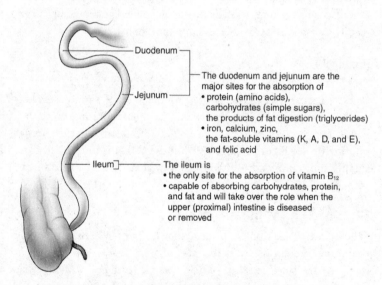

Duodenum

Jejunum

The duodenum and jejunum are the major sites for the absorption of
• protein (amino acids),
  carbohydrates (simple sugars),
  the products of fat digestion (triglycerides)
• iron, calcium, zinc,
  the fat-soluble vitamins (K, A, D, and E),
  and folic acid

Ileum

The ileum is
• the only site for the absorption of vitamin B_{12}
• capable of absorbing carbohydrates, protein, and fat and will take over the role when the upper (proximal) intestine is diseased or removed

Figure 5. Absorption Sites in the Small Intestine

If we eat more than the body needs for energy and efficient cellular function, the nutrients are absorbed and stored—primarily as body fat. The digestive system is designed for survival, and this function can outsmart any diet that supplies more food than the body needs at a given time.

Transport

Once the food components are actively absorbed by the intestinal wall, they are transported into the body. Carbohydrates, protein, and fat are taken up (absorbed) from the lumen and transported across the epithelial cell membranes by different mechanisms. Some food components move across quite easily while others require specialized chemical "porters" that literally bind to the components and "carry" them across the cells of the villi. The villi are full-service providers. They not only supply the enzymes and fluids that break down specific foods, they supply the "porters" that enable the food components to enter the body.

Carbohydrates

Carbohydrates supply the body with the fuel it requires for immediate as well as long-term muscle function and energy. The simple sugars are readily transported across the villi into the bloodstream.

Proteins

Proteins are the building blocks of the body, an essential part of every cell, organ, and system. They are made up of amino acids that are usually strung together in "chains" and held together by *peptide bonds*. Enzymes secreted by the pancreas and from the brush border (microvilli, see Figure 3, page 12) split these chains into smaller and smaller molecules and individual amino acids that can then be absorbed.

Gluten: The Problem Protein

When most people think of protein, they think of meat, fish, eggs, and cheese, but protein is an essential part of many foods. And the protein that gives the small intestine of many people (with and without celiac disease) the most trouble is *gliadin,* the alcohol-soluble portion of *gluten,* which is the protein portion of wheat and several other grains. It contains one fraction—a particularly large (thirty-three amino acids long) peptide chain—that is not readily digested. So despite all the grinding, churning, mixing, and battering of digestion, some proteins remain intact. It is this fraction of gliadin that is thought to cause celiac disease.

Fat

Fat is one of the main building blocks of the body, providing long-term energy stores and the cholesterol we need. Cholesterol is the main component of cell membranes and is needed to maintain the integrity of every cell in the body.

Fat breakdown begins in the mouth and is continued in the stomach, but the actions of enzymes from the pancreas and the liver enable the small intestine to digest most of the fats we eat and absorb and transport them into the bloodstream.

Mineral and Vitamin Digestion

Specific minerals and vitamins are crucial to body growth, function, and metabolism. Even minor deficiencies disrupt body chemistry.

Vitamins are either water or fat *soluble*. Water-soluble vitamins, the B family and C, move across the watery chyme quite easily, either on their own or assisted by special carriers. Fat-soluble vitamins must be *emulsified* to make the trip.

Water, sodium (salt), calcium, iron, potassium, and other trace minerals are readily absorbed in different parts of the small intestine. Most require specialized porters to carry them across the brush border. If the villi are damaged and unable to produce and supply these shuttles, minerals and vitamins cannot be absorbed.

Whatever is left of the chyme in the small intestine—mainly non-digestible fibers and fluid—is then pushed by peristalsis into the colon.

The Colon (Large Intestine)

The colon (large intestine) is about six feet long and the bottom end of the digestive tube. It acts as a receptacle for all the liquid and food products that do not get absorbed and prepares them to be eliminated by dehydrating and solidifying them into fecal matter.

The main function of the colon is the absorption of water. As the food is pushed through the colon about two liters of water is absorbed back into the body. The fecal matter becomes more and more concentrated and then stored until it is eliminated through the *rectum*. The longer it takes to expel feces, the more water is absorbed, making the stool harder and, in turn, more difficult to expel. Diets high in fiber (raw

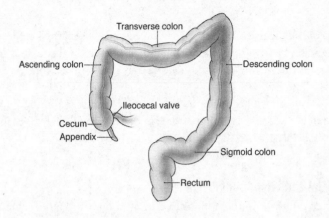

Figure 6. The Large Intestine

fruits and vegetables, high-fiber cereals) create greater fecal bulk that goes largely unabsorbed by the small intestine and creates larger stools.

The colon is also inhabited by a large population of different bacteria that happily dine on and digest the unused fiber from our diet. Because of the slow movement of food in the colon, bacteria have ample time to multiply in this environment. About one-third of fecal matter is bacteria. These bacteria are beneficial because they produce vitamins, such as vitamin K. They also produce gas, a waste product of their own digestive process.

Unlike the small intestine, which is controlled by involuntary muscles (occurring automatically), our brains and extrinsic nerves—facilitated by stress, prunes, and opportunity—play a role in regulating the ano-rectal muscles.

When Normal Goes Pathological

With an understanding of the normal workings of the digestive system, it is easier to comprehend what happens when it gets broken.

If the intestines do not contract properly as in diabetic neuropathy or scleroderma, there is impaired mixing of intestinal contents, which affects digestion and absorption. The lack of movement also means a higher rate of *bacterial overgrowth* (see Chapter 3) that can affect both the digestion and absorption of nutrients.

- You can do without a gallbladder, but a blocked *bile duct,* where bile cannot be released into the small intestine, results in the malabsorption of fats.
- If the pancreas is diseased, there may be no amylase to break up the larger carbohydrate molecules, lipase to break down fat, or trypsin to break down protein. (See Pancreatic Insufficiency, Chapter 16.)
- If the liver is diseased, the bile salts and fluids that digest fat are missing and transport of fats to and through the body is affected.
- If the intestinal villi are inflamed or destroyed, the digestion of food can be altered, disrupted, or completely halted. Food is maldigested and malabsorbed. It remains in the lumen, enters the colon, and causes diarrhea. And malabsorption feeds on itself—the lack of nutrients radiating throughout and eventually affecting the entire body.
- In a diseased state, the amount of fluid getting into the colon can exceed the capacity to absorb it and stool remains liquid. In addition, the products of digestion that were not absorbed (e.g., sugars, bile salts, fatty acids) stimulate the colon to *secrete* water. This causes more diarrhea. When the bacteria colonizing the colon act on the sugars, this can cause distention, cramps, and gas.

In Summary

The digestive system is a wonderfully meshed machine that turns the food we eat into nutrients that support all of the functions and systems of the body. And it is within the small intestine with its enormous absorptive surface that we find the focal point for the ultimate digestion, absorption, and transport of these nutrients. If the intestine is damaged in any way, or in multiple ways, we lose these mechanisms. The body is starved for the nutrients it requires to stay healthy.

Diseases can upset any one, several, or all of the processes of digestion, absorption, transport, secretion, and contraction. Celiac disease is a disease of absorption.

The Digestive Tract in Flames: Celiac Disease

Something deeply hidden had to be behind things.
—From Ralph E. Lapp, The Einstein Letter That Started It All *(1964)*

When the GI tract is functioning normally, we have no perception of digestion. Similarly, we cannot feel our blood circulate or our skin "breathe" unless there is something wrong with those processes. But when digestion is altered or interrupted, when the normal physiology breaks down, we usually know it. Unfortunately, the symptoms may not appear to match the problem.

Celiac Disease

Celiac disease—a multisystem disease in which the gastrointestinal tract is the major site of injury—is one of the most underdiagnosed hereditary autoimmune disorders.

In an autoimmune disease, the body attacks itself. In the case of celiac disease, the body damages or destroys the *villi* (see Figure 4, page 14), the very components of the small intestine that enable us to absorb the nutrients we need to survive. And, much like a domino effect, the damage extends to other parts of the body as it progresses.

The trigger for this destructive reaction is gluten, a group of proteins found primarily in wheat, rye, and barley. For those with celiac disease, the immune system treats gluten as a foreign body and inflames the villi of the small intestine in order to protect the body from the perceived invader. The villi, which enable the body to digest and absorb food, inflame and eventually flatten. This can lead to a serious lack of vital nutrients. In some cases, the progress of the reaction is gradual, in others rapid and dramatic.

While we know what triggers the immune response (gluten), the reasons why the response occurs only in certain genetically predisposed individuals and at varying times in their lives are still unclear.

What Is Gluten?

It's amazing that something as small as gluten can wreak such havoc with the body. (Larry, 62)

Gluten is the term for the storage protein of wheat. Wheat is approximately 10 to 15 percent protein; the remainder is starch. Gluten is what remains after the starch granules are washed from wheat flour. The gluten fraction that is most studied in celiac disease is called gliadin, but there are other proteins that chemically resemble gliadin in rye (*secalins*) and barley (*hordeins*). These proteins are not strictly glutens, but are generally included in the term and are toxic to people with celiac disease. Most of the studies in celiac disease look at gliadin, but it is possible that there are other proteins in gluten to which people are sensitive.

If you look at the grain table, you will see that the grass family has numerous branches. Wheat, rye, and barley—which contain gliadin, secalin, and hordein proteins, respectively—are closely related genetically. They come from similar tribes that also include spelt, kamut, and triticale. Oats are on a different branch, closely related to rice, and are believed to be safe for most people (more than 98 percent) with celiac disease. Rice, corn, millet, sorghum, and several other grains are also safe. (For more on this subject, see Part IV.)

Normally when we digest protein, it gets broken down in the stomach and small intestine into single amino acids or *dipeptides* (two amino acid molecules) that are readily absorbed by the small intestine. But the gluten molecule is resistant to the enzymes that break down proteins (peptidases). It is simply not digested well by humans. As a result, we are left with a long peptide chain, composed of thirty-three amino acids, that is called the toxic fraction of gliadin. This toxic fragment gets into the lining of the intestine, underneath the epithelial

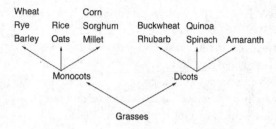

Figure 7. The Grain Families

cells lining the villi. (See Figure 2, page 12.) And some people develop an immunological reaction to this gliadin fraction that starts to inflame and destroy the villi.

The small gluten fragments enter the bowel in both health and disease. It is believed that they enter between as well as through the cells. It may also be related to breaks in the mucosal barrier caused by an infection. It is also unclear how gliadin initiates the immune response and intestinal changes that lead to celiac disease. These areas are the subject of current research into the disease. (See Chapter 27.) What is understood is that the gliadin fraction is the main environmental trigger and culprit in the disease. It only becomes harmful when tissue transglutaminase (tTG) is activated. Essentially, **celiac disease is an abnormal reaction to a normal food substance.**

So, while wheat may be the "staff of life" for some, for others it more closely resembles the "terminator."

What Goes Wrong: The Role of Inflammation

As described in Chapter 1, the digestive system is constantly open to the bacteria, toxins, and foreign elements in our food and water supply. The system's first line of defense is an intact mucosa—the lining of the entire GI tract. The second defense is the actions of gastric acid, which rid the system of many of the unwanted organisms that we might ingest. The third barrier erected by the digestive system is a limited, but constant level of inflammation that is present in the intestine, dealing with the potentially toxic environment. This controlled inflammation is one of the body's initial immune responses and serves to seal off the infected area.

The inflammation is caused by a family of white blood cells that are designed to protect the body from all types of toxins. These white blood cells produce antibodies (*immunoglobulins,* Ig) that target microbes. These immunoglobulins play an important role in helping the body to prevent or to get rid of infections. Of particular interest to the digestive system, IgA (immunoglobulin A) is made in abundance by the intestinal immune system and is secreted into both the lumen of the intestine and the bloodstream. Fetuses receive IgG antibodies from the maternal blood as it crosses the placenta, and breast-fed children receive IgA antibodies through mother's milk. These two sources of antibodies are important forms of protection for infants until their own immune systems have developed.

When working properly, the inflammatory mechanisms and our immunological arsenal allow us to take in nutrients and keep unwanted food toxins, parasites, and bacteria out. But when the body senses an invasion of any kind, it responds to eliminate the problem. The normal level of inflammation increases as more and more inflammatory cells are attracted to the area "under attack." Each cell has a specific job. Many act as messengers, calling for reinforcements. As more "troops" are deployed to the area, damage occurs to the tissue that is being protected.

The body's arsenal consists of a variety of white blood cells and inflammatory messengers that release chemicals to kill bacteria and unwanted materials and attract more inflammatory cells—which continues the inflammatory response. *Macrophages,* the scavenger cells of the immune system, are recruited to clean up the damage. They engulf and destroy foreign matter, but they also liberate more enzymes that cause tissue damage.

It is much like the scene of a fire after water and chemicals have extinguished the blaze and caused their own forms of residual damage. If production of these toxic products continues unchecked, not only are the foreign antigens destroyed, but normal tissues are damaged and normal regrowth and regeneration cannot occur.

The actual substances that cause the damage are the *cytokines,* specifically a cytokine called *interferon gamma.* These protein messengers release chemicals that cause inflammation and flattening of the villi (*villous atrophy*). Villous atrophy is not specific to celiac disease; it is the main way the small intestine responds to any insult. (For more on research into blocking the cytokines as a treatment for celiac disease, see Chapter 27.)

Finally, plasma cells in the inflamed tissue release antibodies in response to the inflammation and assault. These antibodies are specific to the pathogen or toxin they are fighting. By identifying these specific antibodies through blood tests, physicians can then determine the cause(s) and, therefore, the treatments for a disease or infection.

What Is Tissue Transglutaminase (tTG)?

In order to understand what is believed to be one of the key mechanisms that cause celiac disease, it is important to understand the role of *tissue transglutaminase*, or *tTG*. tTG is an important enzyme that is found in every tissue of the body. tTG acts by joining proteins together, a crucial part of wound healing and bone growth. But while tTG is continually acting to protect us, heal wounds, and get rid of damaged tissue, it also acts on gliadin, turning it into a more toxic molecule for people with celiac disease.

It is believed that tTG converts the gliadin molecule into a form that interacts with and activates specific immune cells. This triggers an immune "recognition factor" in certain genetically prone individuals that sets off the inflammatory process that results in damage to the villi. Therefore, to have celiac disease, you need gliadin, tissue transglutaminase, and certain genes.

As part of this interaction with gliadin, tTG gets incorporated into the white blood cells that are making antibodies to fight the inflammation. As a result, these cells produce antibodies to tTG. These antibodies are not thought to be responsible for the damage; they are thought to be a phenomenon that goes along with the process. Therefore, testing for antibodies to tTG is one highly specific way of testing for celiac disease.

The Intestinal Battlefield

When the immune system senses a serious infection or foreign invader, the normally controlled inflammatory process revs up. After repeated assaults, the inflammation causes the villi to atrophy (shrink) and eventually flatten, losing their absorptive power. The loss of the villi reduces the surface area available for absorption and destroys the enzymes in the microvilli responsible for the digestion and transport of nutrients. (Without the epithelial cell barrier, our immune system begins to make more antibodies to food proteins.)

The inflammatory response resembles a battlefield with different troops racing to the scene, releasing their chemical weapons, and leaving a great deal of damage and debris. Much as in any conflict, if there are only occasional skirmishes, there is not much ancillary damage, and the body can repair itself. This happens when we eat spoiled food, get a stomach "bug," drink water with an unfamiliar local bacterium, and so forth. The body responds by putting in more inflammation. The inflammation deals with the problem, and then the body recovers.

In the digestive tract of people with celiac disease, the gliadin molecule gets into the intestinal lining and continually stimulates the inflammatory response. The inflammation becomes excessive and causes continuous damage to the villi until the triggering toxin is removed.

The Digestive Tract in Flames

The digestive tract of people with celiac disease presents a pathological picture of:

- Villous atrophy (flattened villi)
- *Crypt hyperplasia* (the crypts, where the epithelial cells that cover the villi are made, work overtime but ineffectively, creating cells that cannot be used)
- Intense inflammatory reaction

Essentially, the body does not perceive that it is attacking itself, only a "foreign" protein in food. But the immunological reaction destroys the very thing it is trying to protect.

The intestine will not recover until you interrupt the vicious cycle by taking gluten out of the diet. This allows the inflammation to abate and normal intestinal appearance to return. With the regrowth of the villi, function can return. Until then, the digestive system creates symptoms that reflect the level of damage to the body—it begins to ask or yell for help.

Figure 8. Biopsy Slide of Total Villous Atrophy

This biopsy slide was taken from an asymptomatic twenty-one-year-old
female in whom blood tests for celiac disease were positive. They
were taken because her mother was diagnosed with celiac disease.

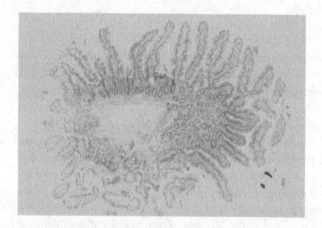

Figure 9. Biopsy Slide of Normal Villi

This normal duodenal biopsy shows long fingerlike villi
with small, short crypts.

(Slides courtesy of Peter H. R. Green, M.D.)

3

How Does Celiac Disease Affect You?

I didn't leave the house for six months; I had to be near the bathroom. (Casey, 34)

I never felt well, and I never felt sick enough to see a doctor. (Marilyn, 28)

The symptoms of celiac disease may come on gradually or they may appear suddenly and dramatically. Symptoms may also wax and wane over a long period of time. Compounding the diagnostic challenge, there are approximately six "silent" or asymptomatic cases for each symptomatic one. Underlying the entire discussion is the medical question of what constitutes a symptom of celiac disease, since the definition is changing and covers a large spectrum of disorders.

My daughter had vomiting and diarrhea starting in February. The pediatrician thought it was gastritis or reflux from February to July. We did neurological scans—he thought the vomiting was neurological, something with her balance. He sent me to a gastroenterologist who thought it looked like gastritis, did barium through the nose (an upper GI). Everything connected to gastritis or reflux.

By July, she had lost eight pounds, lost her hair, and stopped walking. She had no more muscle on her legs. She had that distended belly like a starved child . . . such a skinny neck . . . and she started getting the black rings under her eyes and the black lips and the pediatrician kept saying, "You just have to go through this, a lot of kids vomit and have diarrhea, it's no big deal."

My daughter weighed twenty-five and change at her two-year visit, and five months later, she was sixteen pounds. I told my husband I don't think she's going to make it.

The gastroenterologist discovered the celiac disease four days before we came to the hospital. I was told, "Just give her gluten-free foods, any store will know what you mean, she'll be fine," and he hung up on me. When she stopped moving, we drove in the middle of the night to the hospital and the resident told me if we'd waited a day longer she would have been dead. She was so severely dehydrated and malnourished.

She was hospitalized and needed to stay on the feeding tube for eleven days. We had gotten so far into the disease that her intestines and her gut were just in such disrepair. We had to train her to walk again. I thought she was going to die. We finally took her home and cooked gluten-free foods for her.

After one month, she gained seven pounds, she looked chubby, and her hair was growing in. (Ilyssa, 33)

Celiac disease was once considered a "wasting" disease, specific to early childhood. The typical picture was a child of less than two years of age with malabsorption symptoms, including diarrhea, failure to thrive, muscle wasting, a distended belly (the textbook case), irritability, and sleep disturbance. Ninety percent of children with these symptoms—diarrhea and failure to thrive—are diagnosed with celiac disease within the first five years of life.

Today, studies have shown that the majority of patients do not have "classic" celiac disease but a "silent" presentation. They either have minimal or no gastrointestinal (GI) symptoms, but suffer from related autoimmune diseases, complications from untreated celiac disease and/or the manifestations of malabsorption. Most patients are diagnosed in their fourth to sixth decades of life and have symptoms for approximately nine years prior to diagnosis.

Until the National Institutes of Health (NIH) Consensus Conference in 2004, celiac disease was classified as typical (the classic symptomatology described above) versus atypical (all nondiarrheal symptoms). There, experts from around the world concurred that atypical celiac disease was now the most common form of presentation and changed the medical terminology for the condition. It is hoped that this will also change the perception of the disease in the professional communities and shorten the time frame to diagnosis.

Severe or "Classic"

I realized I had never cut (my daughter's) nails in a year. I thought the nurse was cutting her nails, the nurse thought I was cutting them. In the hospital, going over all her symptoms, we realized no one was cutting them: she had no nail growth. (Ilyssa, 33)

"Classic" celiac disease connotes mild to severe symptoms that predominantly involve the GI tract. The severity of intestinal symptoms is directly related to the amount of intestine that is damaged. Severe cases involve villous atrophy throughout much of the length of the small intestine and malabsorption affecting all nutrients. If the malabsorption is severe, it may result in dramatic weight loss and vitamin deficiency. Severe cases usually result in gastrointestinal disturbances, including diarrhea, cramps, bloating, lactose intolerance, increased reflux, and *dyspepsia*.

Atypical Celiac Disease

The inflammatory process and villous atrophy may involve only the upper part of the GI tract, and may or may not progress very far down the length of the small intestine. People with this condition may malabsorb a single nutrient such as iron or calcium in the proximal (upper) portions of the small intestine. This leads to associated conditions such as anemia, osteopenia, or osteoporosis. Many of these patients also have mild but persistent gastrointestinal symptoms such as reflux, bloating, and dyspepsia that often get labeled as irritable bowel syndrome (IBS).

I was diagnosed in 1991. We had my daughter screened in 1993 because she was so very thin. Her test results were totally negative. In 1997, she was a college senior, at a good weight. To our surprise, she was diagnosed after participating in a family screening study. One of my sons was also tested at that family screening. He had no symptoms and the results were negative, as expected.

A year and a half later, he was screened again as part of a family genetic study. We were all shocked when his antibodies were totally positive.

Both my son and daughter were completely asymptomatic, yet their diagnosis was confirmed with positive biopsy results. I have another son who has recurrent GI (gastrointestinal) problems. He too has been screened twice and biopsied once, all with totally negative results. I was so surprised by the results of my children's screenings that I wrote an article—"Don't Try to Guess Who Is the Celiac in Your Family." (Sue Goldstein, founder of the Westchester Celiac Sprue Support Group)

Silent Celiac Disease

Some patients with silent celiac disease recognize their milder symptoms only retrospectively. The sense of fatigue that comes on after an illness or pregnancy and never seems to dissipate; dental enamel defects that are attributed to antibiotics; childhood irritability and illness.

Some people exhibit no gastrointestinal symptoms due to the celiac disease itself until they develop a complication such as adenocarcinoma (cancer) of the small intestine. Patients also present with diabetes or anemia. Patients with silent celiac disease often appear later in life with symptoms of what are now understood to be related conditions such as dermatitis herpetiformis (an intensely itchy skin condition), peripheral neuropathies (numbness and tingling in the extremities), depression, or infertility.

Because some patients are *truly* asymptomatic, it is important to understand that the malabsorption of nutrients is dangerous to one's general health. Many patients who do not have diarrhea think that there is no need for treatment. But the longer individuals have celiac disease, the more likely they are to get other autoimmune diseases. (See Chapter 14.) **Even without any symptoms, patients need to be treated to prevent further damage.**

Every Body Reacts Differently

It is not clear why some people get dermatitis herpetiformis and others neuropathies or migraines. Each body reacts idiosyncratically to the lack of certain vitamins or minerals as well as to the disease. The long-term effects of celiac disease also range from the silent to the severe.

The four major categories of symptoms and complications are:

1. Intestinal problems (diarrhea, flatulence, reflux, and pain and bloating)

2. The manifestations of malabsorption (vitamin deficiency, iron deficiency, fatigue, calcium malabsorption leading to osteoporosis, and protein and calorie malnutrition causing weight loss and muscle atrophy)

3. Systemic inflammatory reactions and autoimmune diseases

4. Malignancies

Within each of these categories, the manifestations range from very mild to potentially life-threatening—but the reason for this variable expression of the disease is unclear.

Intestinal Problems

Diarrhea

It started as an infant. I had to be on special formulas. I remember having to tell my mother when I made a "frankfurter"—as opposed to the diarrhea I usually had. (Sara, 43)

Diarrhea is most commonly the result of infections, viruses, or toxins due to "food poisoning." This diarrhea is self-limiting—once the body rids itself of the unwanted organisms or toxins, the intestines return to normal.

In celiac disease, the diarrhea may come and go, but it usually recurs. "I had five episodes of gastroenteritis last year" is a common refrain. There are several mechanisms at work.

The Burn. What is going on in the intestines is much like what happens to skin that has been burned. When someone is badly burned, they lose fluid, serum, and protein through the inflamed, destroyed skin layers. When an individual has prolonged inflammation in the intestine, the epithelial cell barrier breaks down and loses its integrity, or barrier function. It is a two-way process—the intestine becomes permeable to substances that would not usually get absorbed, and the barrier to fluid loss is breached. The intestines "weep" or ooze serum (blood fluids). The medical term is *protein-losing enteropathy*. People lose the protein in their blood through weeping of serum. The loss includes that of surface area, villi, and microvilli.

Malabsorption. The second major cause of diarrhea is malabsorption. When sugars and fat are malabsorbed, they draw water into the colon. In a diseased state, the amount of fluid getting into the colon exceeds its capacity to absorb it and the stool remains liquid.

In addition, the products of digestion that were not absorbed (for example, sugars, bile salts, and fatty acids) stimulate the colon to secrete water. The colon loses its function and secretes rather than absorbs liquid.

All of the bacteria that inhabit the colon hungrily dine on the available sugars and fats, releasing gas and causing distention, cramps, and increased flatulence. Malabsorption can occur when any of the organs of the digestive system are diseased and disrupt digestion, absorption, or transport.

When children present with a failure to thrive or with short stature, it is an indication of malabsorption. They get diarrhea more frequently than adults with celiac disease because their digestive tracts are shorter and they have less area to compensate for damage to the mucosa.

Crypt Hypertrophy. Diarrhea can also be contributed to by *crypt hypertrophy*, which causes increased water secretion. Water secretion occurs mainly in the crypts, water absorption in the villi. (See Figure 4, page 14.) There is usually a delicate balance. With the loss of villi and swelling of the crypts, the secretion far outweighs the absorption.

Lactose Intolerance. A *lactase* insufficiency or secondary *lactose intolerance* can cause diarrhea. Lactase, the enzyme that digests milk products, is produced in the microvilli or brush border of the epithelial cells; so if you lose surface area/epithelium, you lose those enzymes. A gluten-free diet will usually restore the enzymes as well as the villi.

Bacteria. *Bacterial overgrowth* is another contributory cause of diarrhea. Patients with celiac disease have more bacteria in their small intestine than usual. The mechanism is unclear but may be disturbed motility (movement in the digestive tract). The bacteria digest the "digesters," the enzymes, contributing to malabsorption and diarrhea. (For more, see Chapter 16.)

Finally, the definition of diarrhea is sometimes questionable. It revolves around the concept of a "normal" bowel movement. The baseline for assessing a problem is what people are used to having. Most people are conditioned to have one per day. Some people are constipated normally. When stools become looser and more frequent than usual, that indicates something is happening—diarrhea.

When stools are liquid, people have the sensation that more stool is waiting to be expelled, but nothing comes out; or more comes out, and the sensation persists. The medical term is *tenesmus*—a feeling of incomplete evacuation. This commonly occurs with colitis and irritable bowel syndrome (IBS), but it can occur with any cause of diarrhea.

Flatulence

> I had no symptoms, but a lot of gas. I thought it was a family trait. My mother and brother had it. (Sandy, 38)

Another common intestinal problem is flatulence. Gas is created by the fermentation of food products in the intestine. It is perfectly normal and generally odiferous, and it's often treated with humor or embarrassment. Doctors who have researched the phenomenon and published data on the subject report that people pass gas (*flatus*), on average, ten times each day, and passage of gas of up to twenty times daily is still considered normal. While this may be more information than some people require, it is important to note that people are more gassy on a high-fiber diet and when they malabsorb sugars, as in lactose intolerance. There is currently no research on how often someone with celiac disease passes gas.

Reflux

> The acid and pain was horrendous; I used to eat Rolaids for dinner. I tried saltines, Cream of Wheat, graham crackers. I was doing myself in—and thinking I was doing the right thing. (Anna, 40)

Reflux, or GERD (gastroesophageal reflux disease), is quite common. It is estimated that 20 percent to 40 percent of the population regularly have heartburn, the most common symptom of reflux. It is the main reason people buy over-the-counter antacids.

People with celiac disease have an increased tendency to get heartburn. This is due to a gastric motility (muscle movement) problem. The stomach does not empty properly and the contents tend to reflux (to flow back up the esophagus). This is aggravated by a reduced lower esophageal sphincter tone (the one-way valve through which food travels from the esophagus into the stomach), which predisposes the stomach contents to reflux. Some patients report that their reflux and heartburn improve on a gluten-free diet.

Pain and Bloating

I would eat a meal and blow up—literally. I looked eight months pregnant. It was like someone pumped me full of gas. Oh, you cannot believe the pain. It got worse when we went to Italy. All that great bread and pasta—I was doubled over. I couldn't button my pants. (Ingrid, 52)

People with excess gas, diarrhea, or reflux experience varying degrees of pain and bloating. They are the classic symptoms of stomach and/or intestinal distress, otherwise known as dyspepsia. They are common signs of lactose intolerance, irritable bowel syndrome, malabsorption, obstruction, and many other intestinal problems. People may experience these symptoms because of celiac disease.

The Manifestations of Malabsorption

While intestinal problems (diarrhea and flatulence) were once considered to be the major manifestations of celiac disease, the more remote effects of malabsorption are now understood to be the most common symptoms seen by doctors.

The ability of the small intestine to compensate for malabsorption in one section is at once remarkable and specifically limited. Fat and sugars are absorbed mainly in the proximal intestine. As explained earlier, when they are malabsorbed, they get into the colon, causing diarrhea. But many people do not get diarrhea because the last third of the small intestine, the ileum, can absorb fats and sugars and can compensate for damage in the duodenum and jejunum.

Vitamins and Minerals

These nutrients are absorbed only in specific sections of the small intestine. Vitamin B_{12} is absorbed in the ileum, so it is not common for people with celiac disease to have vitamin B_{12} malabsorption.

Iron, much of our calcium, fat-soluble vitamins, and folic acid get absorbed in the proximal portion of the small intestine, where celiac disease does much of its damage. Therefore, most people with celiac disease will have bone problems ranging from osteopenia to osteoporosis because of calcium malabsorption, and low *ferritin* (the form that iron takes when stored for usage in the body), indicating iron deficiency.

The potential for vitamin and mineral deficiency is one of the reasons it is important for all patients diagnosed with celiac disease to see a nutritionist/dietician. The chart that follows outlines the fat-soluble vitamins commonly malabsorbed in celiac disease. It also outlines their function and their effect on the body.

FAT-SOLUBLE VITAMINS

Vitamin A
FUNCTION: Plays an essential role in vision and retinal function; necessary for sexual reproduction, normal growth, bone development, growth of epithelial tissue, and the immune system.

Deficiency can cause anemia and reproductive, vision, and growth problems. Severe deficiencies can result in inhibited growth, night blindness, and loss of the sense of taste. Excess amounts of vitamin A can be toxic.

Vitamin D
FUNCTION: Important factor in the intestinal absorption of calcium and bone growth.

Deficiency causes rickets (soft, deformed bones) in children and can contribute to calcium and bone problems (osteopenia and osteoporosis) in adults. Excess amounts can be toxic; supplements should be monitored.

Vitamin E

FUNCTION: An antioxidant that protects cells from damage.

Deficiency has been associated with neurological problems, such as peripheral neuropathy and ataxia, and anemia. There is concern that excess amounts can be toxic.

Vitamin K

FUNCTION: Aids in blood clotting. Anticoagulant drugs such as Coumadin prevent coagulation by blocking the actions of vitamin K.

Deficiency results in impaired synthesis of clotting factors in the liver. In turn, bruising and easy bleeding occur.

The fat-soluble vitamins are absorbed with other fats in the proximal intestine and require bile and pancreatic secretions to be properly digested. They are malabsorbed when the small intestine or interacting organs of digestion (the pancreas, liver, or bile ducts) are impaired. Levels of vitamins A and D can be measured and should be checked if specific symptoms warrant a closer inspection.

Anemia

> For years I was anemic. Doctors said: "You have your period, you don't eat right." So, I would take iron and it would make me sick. I was constipated and having abdominal pain. There were points I couldn't take it anymore. (Lori, 31)

The body stores iron in the liver and bone marrow as a molecule called ferritin. Iron is extremely important to the body, helping to carry oxygen in the blood and aiding in energy production, cellular respiration, and immune function. When iron stores are depleted—due to blood loss and/or malabsorption—and not replaced through the diet, you become anemic. The consequences have a large impact on bodily function.

There are three kinds of anemia:

- Microcytic (small red blood cells; most often due to iron deficiency)

- Normocytic (red cells normal size; most often due to chronic illness and inflammation)

- Macrocytic (red cells larger than normal; most often due to vitamin B_{12} or folic acid deficiency)

Anemia in celiac disease can be caused by multiple factors including iron deficiency, folate (folic acid) deficiency, vitamin B_{12} deficiency, and chronic inflammation.

The most common cause of anemia in women is menstrual blood loss. In men, it is blood loss through injury or an intestinal problem. People suffering from persistent anemia, especially iron deficiency anemia, where other underlying medical conditions have been ruled out, should ask their doctors about testing for celiac disease.

Fatigue

I was so exhausted I couldn't leave the house, I couldn't walk. My father thought I had Lyme disease. (Heather, 43)

Fatigue is one of the major complaints of people with celiac disease. It is also seen in numerous other medical conditions; therefore, many doctors look elsewhere for a diagnosis.

Nevertheless, extreme fatigue has a true physiological basis as one of the major side effects of celiac disease.

Fatigue can be caused by:

- Malnutrition and the malabsorption of nutrients

- Inflammation in the intestines (inflammation in any location causes fatigue; see Inflammation, Chapter 7)

- Iron deficiency (anemia is a potential contributory factor)

- Vitamin, folic acid, and B_{12} deficiency

- Carnitine deficiency (an amino acid that can be supplemented if blood tests indicate low levels)

- Assorted autoimmune disorders such as thyroid problems

- Depression

After ruling out other physical and/or psychological causes, chronic fatigue should be considered as a symptom of celiac disease. (See discussion of chronic fatigue syndrome, Chapter 5.)

Osteoporosis

Calcium is the most abundant mineral in the body, and most of it is stored in skeletal bone. When calcium is malabsorbed, bones become demineralized and eventually porous.

Osteoporosis, literally "porous bone," is a disease in which bones become so fragile that the skeleton is unable to sustain the body's weight and the stresses of normal activity. It is a "silent" condition because most people do not know they have thin bones until one of them breaks. Low bone density and osteoporosis are common in patients with celiac disease. Low blood calcium levels are a specific marker for the condition. (For a specific discussion of osteoporosis in celiac disease, see Chapter 9.)

Neuropathies

Some neuropathies (a condition caused by the inflammation of nerves) can be caused by a deficiency of vitamin B_{12} or E, but they are more commonly autoimmune. (For a specific discussion of the neuropathies related to celiac disease, see Chapter 7.)

Systemic Inflammatory Reactions and Autoimmune Diseases

While malabsorption underlies many of the symptoms of celiac disease, the inflammatory process itself is now understood to be a major factor in the development of symptoms. Inflammation, mainly through the increased levels of circulating cytokines, makes people feel unwell.

It is well documented that autoimmune diseases tend to travel in tandem. That is, if you develop one, you are more likely to develop another. It is believed that this is most likely due to a genetic predisposition. Approximately 8 to 10 percent of all type 1 diabetics have celiac disease, and the number may be higher as more patients are diagnosed. Among the patients seen at the Celiac Disease Center at Columbia, 30 percent have at least one associated autoimmune disorder, compared with 3 percent of the general population.

People with one diagnosed autoimmune disease and unexplained symptoms should explore the link with celiac disease.

Malignancies

People with celiac disease have a twofold greater chance to develop a malignancy than the general population. The malignancies that occur at an increased rate are mainly lymphomas, but also include esophageal carcinoma, small intestinal adenocarcinoma, and non-Hodgkin's lymphoma. A gluten-free diet appears to reduce the risk of developing these malignancies to that of the general population after five years of compliance—with the exception of non-Hodgkin's lymphoma. (For more on this subject, see Chapter 8.)

Celiac disease has been dubbed the "great pretender." Its protean symptoms and systemic manifestations can easily masquerade as a number of other illnesses. And it is those conditions that are often diagnosed instead of celiac disease. The one thing most patients have in common is a long road to diagnosis.

4

How Do I Know If I Have It?
The Diagnosis of Celiac Disease

*I finally told my umpteenth doctor: I don't want another Band-Aid.
I want you to cure me!* (Gene, 49)

*My two-year-old son went from the 97th percentile of the growth
chart to the 23rd and the pediatrician said we were a small family,
he was probably just small....* (Enid, 35)

Despite the growing awareness of celiac disease, the road to diagnosis
can still be long and bumpy. The celiac iceberg hides under a sea of
symptoms and manifestations that can confuse both doctor and patient.

Celiac disease is alternatively called by some professionals an allergy, sensitivity, or intolerance. While some of the symptoms are similar, it is important to distinguish among them.

Food Allergy versus Gluten Intolerance
versus Food or Non-Celiac Gluten Sensitivity

An *antigen* is defined as any foreign material that triggers an immune
response in our body. Until a baby's immune system develops, most
foods are "foreign material." Breast milk or a substitute formula is the
first food. Breast milk is more easily tolerated by immature immune
systems and provides antibodies to the child. Fruits, vegetables, meats,
and so forth eventually replace formula so that a baby's immune system

can slowly acclimate to different external substances coming into his or her body. At some stage in this process, some susceptible people develop allergies, intolerances, and/or sensitivities to specific foods or substances. A food that is tolerated by most people may become an antigen and trigger an immune response in another person.

Food Allergies

These are a common type of immunological reaction in which the body produces antibodies in response to specific foods. In Chapter 2 we discussed the immune arsenal and the role of antibodies (immunoglobulins, Ig) in protecting the body against bacteria and viruses. Of the different types of antibodies, *immunoglobulin E, IgE,* is the main concern if you are allergic. It is the IgE antibodies that circulate throughout our bloodstream and trigger the *immediate* immune response that is an "allergic reaction."

IgE antibodies are formed when the immune system recognizes a substance as an antigen. When it "sees" the antigen again, it causes the release of chemicals such as histamines, which produce symptoms that may include swelling, asthma, itching, inflammation, vomiting, diarrhea, respiratory distress, and shock. The presence of IgE antibodies in the blood is suggestive of a food allergy.

Allergic reactions are immediate, occurring within seconds or up to several hours.

Celiac disease is a delayed type of immune reaction—it is not a food allergy.

Gluten Intolerance

Gluten intolerance is a widely used and often misconstrued label. By definition, if you have celiac disease, you are gluten intolerant. But, it is possible to be gluten intolerant and not have celiac disease. Anyone who has symptoms brought on by the ingestion of gluten that are relieved by its removal from the diet can be called gluten intolerant. Some irritable bowel syndrome (IBS) symptoms are relieved by gluten withdrawal; those individuals are gluten intolerant.

Many people are given this "diagnosis" based on lay information. Or some people will diagnose themselves out of frustration at a lack of medical consensus as to what is causing their symptoms.

The "gold standard" for diagnosing celiac disease is still the intestinal biopsy (see page 47), and that is recommended for individuals contemplating a gluten-free diet for the rest of their lives. **Celiac disease is a serious medical condition that should not be self-diagnosed.**

Non-Celiac Gluten Sensitivity

Non-celiac gluten sensitivity is another catchall term. If you have celiac disease, you are by definition gluten sensitive. But it is often used to describe patients who do not have celiac disease. When a patient has a specific food sensitivity, all symptoms go away when the offending food is removed from the diet.

Recent studies and clinical observation are showing that non-celiac gluten sensitivity may be much more common than previously thought. It may, in fact, be a separate disease entity that involves different organs and different mechanisms than celiac disease. While there is no doubt that the condition exists, the lack of definite criteria for a diagnosis has resulted in a skeptical attitude on the part of many doctors. Patients have therefore sought out nonmedical practitioners and labs offering often questionable answers and results.

The acceptance of non-celiac gluten sensitivity as a valid condition has evolved. Patients with irritable bowel syndrome and various neurological conditions have improved while on a gluten-free diet. (See Chapter 7.) Research has shown that patients with dermatitis herpetiformis have increased antibodies to epidermal transglutaminase (tTG3), which is different from—but part of the family of—the tTG involved in celiac disease (tTG2). (See What Is Tissue Transglutaminase [tTG]?, Chapter 2.) Similarly, patients with gluten-sensitive neurological syndromes have antibodies to tTG6. It is therefore possible that a separate immune mechanism is at work with non-celiac gluten sensitivity. It is probably multiple conditions.

We define non-celiac gluten sensitivity as patients with symptoms that improve when gluten is removed from their diet and relapse on reintroduction.

Non-celiac gluten sensitivity, as a diagnostic term, should be reserved for those individuals who have a normal intestinal biopsy and a predictable and recurring set of symptoms relieved by removing gluten from the diet.

Therefore, if you get sick when ingesting gluten, you may be gluten sensitive and may benefit from a gluten-free diet.

Many of the symptoms of celiac disease can and do occur in other conditions. When all is explored and examined, physicians need to rely on blood and pathology tests to confirm a diagnosis. The presence of normal test results often makes it difficult to get a diagnosis.

The Diagnosis

The only definitive means of accurately diagnosing celiac disease is an intestinal biopsy, the gold standard for diagnosis. While nothing in medicine is 100 percent, this is still considered the most definitive diagnosis. However, specific blood tests (serological testing) are an important indication of whether or not you have celiac disease and a means for the doctor to determine if you should have a biopsy.

Clinical judgment also plays an important role in this diagnosis. If a patient is obviously sick with symptoms that strongly indicate celiac disease, and blood and biopsy tests are negative or inconclusive, tests should be reviewed and/or repeated. Patients are (usually) not doctors, but they know how their bodies feel and function. Labs and professionals can make diagnostic errors, and it is sometimes necessary to push for reconfirmation of a negative test—or get another opinion.

Potential Celiac Disease

There is also a group of people who appear to have potential celiac disease. They may have positive blood tests and a negative biopsy, or negative blood tests that do not warrant a biopsy. This is often seen in first-degree relatives of patients with celiac disease or patients with other autoimmune diseases, especially diabetes and thyroiditis. There is a general acceptance among medical professionals studying celiac disease that potential celiac disease should not be treated with a gluten-free diet. It can mask a wheat sensitivity, place healthy persons on a strict, lifelong diet they need not adhere to, and/or confuse test results conducted at a later date. Treatment should be reserved for those diagnosed with celiac disease. An exception to this may be when patients have symptoms that a physician feels warrant the use of a gluten-free diet. If followed for up to twelve years, only 30 percent of people with potential celiac disease actually develop celiac disease—i.e., villous atrophy.

Blood Tests

There are blood tests that are very specific and sensitive for the diagnosis of celiac disease.

The panel of blood tests available as a first-line indicator of celiac disease includes:

1. IgA tissue transglutaminase antibodies (tTG)—the mainstay of diagnosis; a highly specific and sensitive marker for celiac disease

2. IgA endomysial antibodies (EMA)—a highly specific marker for celiac disease when performed in a high-quality lab

3. Total IgA antibodies—will identify patients who are IgA deficient (see Selective IgA Deficiency, page 46)

4. IgA and IgG deamidated gliadin peptides (DGP)—may reveal celiac disease when positive in setting of negative IgA tTG test

A panel of tests is usually performed because there is no one test that is sensitive and specific enough to pick up everyone with celiac disease. The available panels usually include two or more of the above tests. The list of tests changes as new ones are developed and we become more aware of the advantages and limitations of each test.

We have not included the older generation of antigliadin antibodies (AGA) in the panel because they are not currently available commercially. They have been replaced by the newer-generation gliadin peptide or deamidated gliadin peptide antibody. We have seen patients with celiac disease who have positive AGA (DGP) and negative IgA tTG tests and vice versa.

Sensitivity and Specificity

Testing criteria are based on the sensitivity and specificity of the test. These terms are often used in the medical literature, so it is important to understand their meaning.

Specificity: If a test is 100 percent specific, it means there is nothing else—no other medical condition—that can cause the positive result.

Sensitivity: If a test is 100 percent sensitive, it means that everyone with the disease has a positive test.

Currently, there are no tests that are 100 percent specific and 100 percent sensitive for celiac disease, but individual tests have extremely high accuracy. Some blood tests correlate to the degree of villous atrophy; others may be affected by IgA deficiency or other conditions that also display the specific immunological markers being tested.

IgA Endomysial Antibodies (EMA)

Testing for EMA is highly specific, virtually 100 percent so, and about 90 percent sensitive. If this test is positive, it means that virtually 100 percent will have celiac disease, though some patients with celiac disease may not be positive for EMA. Nevertheless, these antibodies correlate to the degree of villous atrophy. (See Selective IgA Deficiency, page 46.)

This is a test done using immunofluorescence technique. It is expensive and is read manually by a technician using a microscope. Therefore, it is observer-dependent, which introduces an element of potential technician error.

The tTG and EMA may be intermittently positive in some individuals. (See Potential Celiac Disease, page 43.) EMA and IgA tTG may also be absent in patients younger than two years of age. In this age group the gliadin peptide antibody may be more significant. This emphasizes the importance of having a biopsy to confirm the diagnosis.

Serologic tests, in clinical practice, often lack the sensitivity reported in the medical literature.

IgA Tissue Transglutaminase (tTG)

tTG is the enzyme that converts gliadin into a more toxic molecule. It is generally agreed to be one of the key serologic markers for celiac disease.

Yet, the tTG antibody is not 100 percent specific—there are other causes of its being positive, and they include diabetes, Crohn's disease, and liver disease. Also, people who have celiac disease can have a negative tTG test.

This is an automated test. It is an ELISA—an enzyme-linked immunosorbent assay—that is machine read from a kit that the lab buys. The kit contains the *substrate* to which the blood sample is added—in this case usually human tissue transglutaminase. This process sets off a reaction that is interpreted by a machine as a number that falls into a positive or negative range.

The test is done with different kits at different laboratories, and results may vary. (See Laboratory Differences, below.)

Deamidated Gliadin Peptides (DGP)

Patients with celiac disease create antibodies to gliadin, but these antibodies can also be found in other conditions and in normal people. It is known that tTG *deamidates*, that is, it acts on and enhances the gliadin peptide in patients with celiac disease, which causes the inflammatory reaction in the gut. These tests have similar sensitivities and specificity as tTG IgA antibody tests. They are often added to the tTG IgA test as a "celiac panel." The addition of DGP increases the diagnosis by about 10 percent. These cases are people with a positive DGP and a negative tTG. However, not all patients with positive DGPs have celiac disease.

Selective IgA Deficiency

There is a genetically determined condition called selective IgA deficiency that occurs in about 0.2 percent of the population and in about 3 percent of patients with celiac disease. These people do not make IgA antibodies, including the IgA celiac antibodies.

Since most of the highly specific and sensitive blood tests for celiac disease measure IgA, the tests are measuring a class of antibody that some people cannot ever make even if the disease is present. Therefore, if a patient's total IgA is below the level of detection, an IgG tissue transglutaminase antibody or gliadin peptide DGP IgG is recommended.

Laboratory Differences

Different labs use different kits to conduct blood tests. These kits have varying normal ranges and various sensitivities and specificities. All of the kits use human tTG as one of the components (either recombinant tTG or tTG from human red cells). However, these different sources of tTG may affect the performance of the test. That is, different kits may give conflicting results on the same blood sample. Therefore, lab results may be positive from one source and negative from another. In addition, all kits may have false positives and negatives. While doctors must rely on serological results from experienced labs, the potential for error and/or the need for repeat blood tests must be understood.

False Negatives/False Positives

Studies have shown that:

- You can have celiac disease and still have negative blood tests. (These patients may have less flattening of the villi and are often harder to identify and diagnose.)
- You can have negative blood tests and develop celiac disease later in life. This is why it is valuable for family members to have the genetic tests. This can determine if an individual has any risk for the development of the disease and should have blood tests done at intervals.
- If you are not ingesting much gluten, your antibodies can be negative and you can still have active celiac disease.

None of the serological tests are either 100 percent specific or 100 percent sensitive for celiac disease, nor are they the clinical standard for diagnosis. Therefore, if the antibodies are negative and the clinical suspicion is high, a biopsy is needed to determine the diagnosis. And if symptoms persist, repeat testing may be indicated.

Tests may also be positive for certain antibodies and indicate another medical condition.

Endoscopy and Biopsy (the Gold Standard for Diagnosis)

Generally, doctors conduct a biopsy when blood tests are positive, if the patient has requested one because of a family diagnosis of celiac disease, or if they have an associated condition such as diabetes and blood tests indicate celiac disease. Many doctors go directly to biopsy when there is a high clinical suspicion—if symptoms, family history, and related conditions strongly point to celiac disease.

Endoscopy is a procedure in which a flexible tube (a scope) is passed down the throat, through the stomach, and into the small intestine so that the doctor can both visualize and biopsy (take a small sample of) the areas. It is generally an outpatient procedure. In the United States people are sedated for the procedure; in some parts of the world they are not.

Patients fast for eight hours so that the stomach is empty. An IV (intravenous line) is put in for sedation. Typically, a local anesthetic spray is used to reduce the gag reflex. The procedure takes ten to twenty minutes.

The procedure is conducted under conscious sedation, which is different from general anesthesia. In general anesthesia, your respiration is suppressed and you are ventilated to help you breathe. With conscious sedation, people remain responsive to commands and their respiration is typically not suppressed. The medication is short-acting and does not take away your vital functions. But the drugs have an amnesiac effect, so people do not experience or remember any discomfort.

Under certain circumstances, people will be given antibiotics prior to the endoscopy. Patients with a preexisting abnormality of the heart or who have had a valve replacement are at higher risk for infection of the valve.

Endoscopy is usually done by a gastroenterologist and a nurse, but anesthesiologists increasingly administer sedation. During the procedure, doctors view the larynx, the esophagus, the stomach, and the duodenum. In order to diagnose celiac disease, they take a duodenal biopsy. The esophagus or stomach is also biopsied if it looks abnormal, or if the patient has symptoms that indicate a problem there. As in any medical procedure, complications can occur, although they are very uncommon.

The lining of the intestine has no pain fibers, so the procedure is painless. There is no risk of bleeding from a routine biopsy because the small amount of oozing stops spontaneously.

How Specific Is a Biopsy?

There are other causes of a positive biopsy—i.e., flattened villi—besides celiac disease. These include HIV disease, tropical sprue, giardiasis, Crohn's disease, a medication reaction (see Drugs That Mimic Celiac Disease, Chapter 5), and even gastroenteritis. These false-positive causes must be ruled out by a physician.

The physician may also biopsy sections of the mucosa that are normal and may "miss" the celiac disease. As we mentioned, celiac disease does not necessarily cause uniform damage—it is "patchy." Therefore, the gastroenterologist takes multiple pieces to increase the chance of finding any abnormality, although failure to take the recommended number of pieces is common. If missed, it can be picked up on a second biopsy. It is always worthwhile having questionable results reviewed by experienced GI pathologists.

The intestinal biopsy is currently the gold standard for the diagnosis of celiac disease. It has been questioned by some experts who feel that the IgA endomysial antibodies (EMA) blood tests are specific enough to confer a positive diagnosis. (This does not apply to other blood tests like the antigliadin and tTG tests, which are *not* specific for celiac disease.) However, we feel that *no* blood test is absolutely 100 percent definitive and that, before one undergoes a permanent diet change, the diagnosis should be as definitive as possible. The biopsy is also needed as a baseline against which to compare further biopsies that may be necessary if a patient does not respond well to a gluten-free diet.

> *It's very important to stress to parents the importance of a biopsy. Psychologically, if you don't have that piece of paper, if the doctor doesn't hold up that slide and say: "Your child has intestinal damage," parents will constantly question the diagnosis.*
>
> *Because once that child is put on the gluten-free diet, he or she will thrive. And then you say: "Maybe Susie isn't celiac." Susie's ten and you give her a little piece of cake and she's fine. And she goes through that little honeymoon period. Then later in her life she may have difficulty getting pregnant, or maybe she's not getting her period. I don't say that happens all the time, but it's very important for parents to know—their child is celiac, this is what your child has. (Elaine Monarch, Celiac Disease Foundation)*

Although many parents do not want to subject their children to an endoscopy and biopsy, their concerns must be weighed against the possibility of an incorrect diagnosis. Parents need to be very sure of the diagnosis prior to embarking with their children on the rigorous, lifelong diet required in celiac disease. At various stages in their lives—starting or changing schools, going to college, traveling—there will be pressure on both parent and child to go off the diet. You need to be very certain of the diagnosis to stay the course.

Finally, it is important to note that a normal biopsy does not necessarily exclude celiac disease for life. Patients with positive endomysial antibodies (EMA) and relatives of patients with celiac disease may harbor a potential form of celiac disease that may appear later in life.

New European Standards for Children

There are pediatric guidelines in Europe that suggest that you can diagnose celiac disease without a biopsy. They are not accepted in the United States. They were created in response to parents' reluctance to subject children to a biopsy that is usually conducted under general anesthesia. If used, these guidelines require very strict protocols that need to be adhered to. The European guidelines require *all* of the following:

The child **must be symptomatic** and then have:

1. A positive tTG more than ten times the upper level of normal
2. A second blood test for EMA that is positive and that *must* be taken on a separate occasion
3. The presence of genetic markers

The second blood draw guards against temporary gluten autoimmunity and may account for "false positive" antibody tests. When these criteria are met, a presumptive diagnosis can be made and a gluten-free diet started.

There are pros and cons to these guidelines. On one hand, most cases of celiac disease are diagnosed by following the guidelines. It eliminates an invasive endoscopy and biopsy, as well as the concern about general anesthesia, which has been suggested as a contributing factor to some cognitive impairment in the very young. However, these detrimental effects on the very young have not been conclusively demonstrated.

Conversely, the guidelines must be adhered to strictly, and some doctors do not do a separate blood draw. It may not catch children who are asymptomatic. Without an endoscopy, other conditions that occur with celiac disease may be missed. And some children with positive blood tests may not have celiac disease.

We favor the certainty of a biopsy since, as the child becomes an adolescent, then an adult, he or she or their adult physician may not believe the diagnosis.

Skin Biopsy

People with dermatitis herpetiformis, the skin manifestation of celiac disease, are diagnosed by a biopsy of the skin immediately adjacent to the erupted blister. **If you have a skin biopsy and it is positive for dermatitis herpetiformis, you do not need to have an intestinal biopsy—you have a confirmed diagnosis of celiac disease.**

Gluten Challenge

A key consideration for all of the tests described is whether the patient has been consuming gluten before being tested. Results of all of the tests will return to normal on a gluten-free diet. Therefore, a gluten challenge—which consists of eating gluten-filled foods for anywhere from one to three months—is often needed in order to confirm a diagnosis of celiac disease. A gluten challenge involves a biopsy, not blood tests, after a period of eating gluten.

There are three major reasons to conduct a gluten challenge:

1. Some people go on a gluten-free diet prior to diagnosis. This is one of the biggest hurdles to accurately assessing a patient with celiac disease. Some people are advised by a doctor, dietician, or friend to do it on a trial basis to see if their symptoms will get better. Other people may live in a household in which family members are gluten-free and thus do not have much gluten in their regular diet. Whatever the reason, people must be ingesting gluten for the tests to be significant.

    If you have stopped eating gluten before having blood work and/or an endoscopy, your doctor should be informed and you should have a gluten challenge before being tested.

2. Some patients do not have definitive results. If the pathology is ambiguous and the doctor has doubts about the diagnosis, a gluten challenge may be indicated.

3. Small children may have a food or cow's milk sensitivity causing the inflammation.

A gluten challenge will clear up any ambivalence regarding the cause.

Many people ask: "How long do I have to eat gluten to have an abnormal blood test?" There is no uniform standard for what a gluten challenge involves. Some literature shows that small amounts of gluten do not elevate blood tests. And some people do not relapse for more than a year. There is no literature on the use of blood tests for a gluten challenge; a biopsy needs to be performed at the end of the challenge.

The standard set by Michael Marsh, M.D., from England, and a long-standing expert in celiac disease*, recommends that a gluten challenge consist of eating about four slices of bread per day for a month. The thought is that most people will show an abnormal biopsy in that amount of time if they have a problem. We now know that a smaller amount of bread over a shorter period of time will result in relapse in most people who have celiac disease. If people are tolerating the gluten well, we would prefer that they remain on gluten for at least three months before having a biopsy. This will reduce the chances that the biopsy result will not be definitive.

The biopsy results for most people on a gluten-free diet will not normalize for six to twelve months, so it is possible to biopsy people within that time frame without a gluten challenge. However, if the biopsy is normal, you cannot definitively conclude whether or not you have celiac disease.

Some patients will say, "I'm not going to ingest gluten, no matter what you tell me; it makes me too sick." That is fine—but you will never be definitively sure if you do or do not have celiac disease. This is an area where genetic testing may be helpful. (See Chapter 17.)

The gluten challenge is an area of controversy. For one, people with positive blood tests and an inconclusive biopsy often do well on a gluten-free diet, and some health care professionals consider this a positive enough diagnosis of celiac disease. But the results from a gluten-free diet are neither sensitive nor specific enough for a diagnosis of celiac disease.

People with non-celiac gluten sensitivity do well on a gluten-free

---

* Marsh MN. Gluten, major histocompatibility complex, and the small intestine. A molecular and immunobiologic approach to the spectrum of gluten sensitivity ("celiac sprue"). *Gastroenterology*. 1992;102(1):330–54.

diet, and many consider this a positive diagnosis of celiac disease. It is not. Finally, patients who have started a gluten-free diet may not show positive blood or biopsy tests for an extended period of time when undertaking a gluten challenge. In addition, a gluten challenge may be dangerous for some patients because the reaction may be severe.

From a medical point of view, it is important that anyone with suspected celiac disease have either repeat blood tests and/or a biopsy to confirm the diagnosis *prior* to their going on a gluten-free diet so that a gluten challenge is not necessary.

Finger Prick Tests

Newer, simpler diagnostic blood tests that only require a drop of blood taken from a finger stick (especially desirable for children) are continually being developed. There are currently a number of home finger prick tests for different conditions. They may seem attractive and inexpensive but results should be interpreted with caution.

The finger stick assay tests for antitissue transglutaminase (tTG) antibodies and is actually conducted in the tube that draws the blood up after a finger stick. It recognizes anti-tTG antibodies. These tests are good in that they detect the same antibodies as whole blood drawn from a vein. They are also subject to the same problems of false positive and negative results.

The finger stick assay is being marketed in parts of Europe and in Canada for use in both the physician's office for diagnosis and as a home test to monitor dietary compliance.

Like any medical test, these tests require interpretation and have varying degrees of sensitivity and specificity. In the doctor's office, they provide an inexpensive point-of-service test. If positive, the patient would then be referred to a gastroenterologist. It therefore raises the issue of what people using the test at home will do with the information provided. Ideally, they will see a doctor, since any diagnosis or treatment should not be undertaken without consulting with a medical professional.

The place for these tests in the diagnosis and management of celiac disease has yet to be definitively determined. However, they appear to be reliable point-of-service screening tests and measure the same antibodies examined when whole blood is drawn. Hopefully, they will increase the diagnosis rate of celiac disease.

Fecal Test

A number of studies have shown that it is possible to recover antibodies from feces. Most of the studies were done on people prior to a colonoscopy after a laxative was taken to wash the intestinal contents through the digestive tract. Studies comparing "normals" and people with celiac disease have shown that these tests are neither sensitive nor specific enough for the diagnosis. Fecal testing is *not* an accepted test for the diagnosis of celiac disease.

There is lay literature on fecal testing that specifically states that the test is an indication of "gluten sensitivity," not that patients have celiac disease. There have not been any studies published in the medical literature that supports this claim.

Saliva Testing

There are now saliva tests available for celiac disease, which offer an interesting alternative to blood tests for young children. Several medical studies have been conducted on their effectiveness, and the literature indicates that salivary tests are currently not sensitive enough to be reliable in diagnosing people with celiac disease. Blood tests are also required as a follow-up, which eliminates some of the appeal of the saliva test.

Research has shown that there can be a discrepancy between blood and saliva concentrations of IgA-AGA, suggesting that systemic and salivary IgA-AGA responses may be controlled separately.

This is an area that requires more study before saliva testing can be considered a first-line option.

Breath Tests

Breath tests are not used to test for celiac disease, but they are a useful, noninvasive tool to assess ongoing symptoms in patients with celiac disease and assess specific problems in the small intestine. (See Chapter 16.) Patients can be tested for lactose intolerance, bacterial overgrowth, fructose and sucrose intolerance, and intestinal transit time.

The test measures the hydrogen gas released from the lungs, a normal by-product of digestion. Patients are given different sugars (sucrose, glucose, lactulose, fructose), and their breath is measured every half hour in order to measure the "peaks" of hydrogen. An increase in hydrogen indicates specific intestinal problems.

Genetic Testing

Genetic testing is not used to diagnose celiac disease. (See Genetic Testing, Chapter 17.)

Nevertheless, it is now available to determine ancestry and some companies give genetic results for medical conditions. It is important to remember that there are multiple factors in addition to genetic makeup that will lead to celiac disease. The presence of specific human leukocyte antigen (HLA) genes is not a determinant of celiac disease, only an indication of an at-risk state. People should *NOT* have a genetic test unless they understand the significance of the test.

Glutenostics–Gluten Detective Rapid Urine/Stool Test

The Gluten Detective urine/stool test is a test designed to detect gluten peptides in the stool or urine. The urine test reflects gluten ingestion in the prior day while the stool test reflects gluten ingested in the previous two to six days.

These tests are accurate and reflect ingested gluten in both the stool and urine of normal, non-celiac individuals as well as those with celiac disease. A recent clinical study from Canada detected gluten in people with celiac disease who were on a strict gluten-free diet. If this test is used as a parameter of strictness, this research suggests that it is very difficult to be on a strict gluten-free diet.

The product is available to the public online as an over-the-counter item (i.e., it does not require a prescription). There are a number of scenarios where patients may wish to buy and use the kits. They include:

- People who have consistently abnormal blood tests or abnormal biopsies might want to use them to document when and where they are getting gluten.
- People who feel that they frequently get contaminated with gluten when eating out. They can test their urine or stool after symptoms occur to see if it is really gluten that is causing them.

The role in the management of celiac disease that these self/home tests play has not been determined. They have come on the market without rigorous FDA studies to determine if there is any benefit of their use. Some people may feel better using these tests, but for others they may cause increased anxiety. We would advise people who use the Gluten Detective tests to discuss the results with their dietician or gastroenterologist. (For gluten testing of food, see The Nima Device, Chapter 21.)

The Future of Testing

In various European countries, national health plans conduct random testing and research in conjunction with the medical community. Many physicians feel that population studies in the United States will uncover the celiac iceberg and help the numerous people who suffer unnecessarily from celiac disease and its related conditions. It is hoped that, with expanded and sophisticated testing, more people will be diagnosed sooner.

The screening tests for celiac disease are constantly being examined in order to understand and increase their specificity, sensitivity, and ease of use. The use of noninvasive diagnostic tools is particularly desirable for the pediatric population.

Since a confirmed diagnosis of celiac disease may prevent serious complications, yet requires a lifelong adherence to a strict gluten-free diet, we feel it is extremely important that the diagnosis is both rapid and correct.

5

Differential Diagnosis: Why Is Celiac Disease Underdiagnosed?

Remedies are our great analyzers of disease.

—Peter Latham

It started as an infant—I had diarrhea and had to be on special formulas. I got my period at fifteen, kind of late. In college, I had symptoms again. I had tests and they ruled out Crohn's disease and diagnosed IBS (irritable bowel syndrome). In medical school, there was a resident doing a platelet (blood) study, and I was supposed to be one of the normal controls. My platelet count was elevated (indicative of iron deficiency as well as celiac disease), and I was anemic. I took iron. By the end, I was taking liquid iron four times a day for a year.

When I got married, my liver function test was slightly elevated. I was told it was okay to get pregnant, and my pregnancy went well, but afterward I became anemic again. I went to a gastroenterological specialist who didn't see clinical signs of liver disease. Then, I went to a liver specialist who thought it was odd that I ate as much as I wanted and never gained any weight. They did thyroid tests and all were normal. I also saw a cardiologist because I had no cholesterol—it was 117.

I'm 5'3" and 108 pounds. I was eating all the time—at work people were jealous. I had no symptoms, but a lot of gas: I thought it was a family trait. I would have diarrhea every now and then, and I would eat rice and bananas and it normalized. When I developed knee pain, I went to an orthopedic specialist and the X-ray showed decreased bone density. I was in my late thirties and thought that was odd. I attributed it to running outside on pavement.

I got really sick during Passover—I always got sick during Passover. I ate a lot of matzo, which was supposed to make you constipated; in my case it caused diarrhea. I went to a gastroenterologist who thought I had picked up a parasite at the hospital (I'm an anesthesiologist). The tests were negative.

I finally looked in an old medical textbook and read the paragraph on celiac disease. I called the gastroenterologist and told him. My husband is a physician and I read him the paragraph. He said: "You would have lost a lot of weight. No one at forty-three has celiac disease."

I was actually a typical case. They did the bloods and I was strongly positive, elevated liver function, anemic. I had the biopsy and had an almost complete loss of villi.

I am a doctor, living in a major city and working at a major hospital. I saw some of the best specialists in each area and no one put it all together. (Sara, 43)

Celiac disease is underdiagnosed for reasons that might be dubbed the three "P's": perception, presentation, and practice.

Perception. Until recently, doctors perceived celiac disease as rare. Part of this is self-fulfilling: If doctors think something is rare, they will not go looking for it. Therefore, they will not find it, and so it remains "rare." If a condition is considered common, doctors will routinely test for it.

Presentation. The disease has changed presentation. The old medical textbooks described celiac disease as a "wasting" disease characterized by diarrhea and malabsorption. But most people do not have diarrhea because of the shift to the "silent" form of celiac disease in the United States. Before 1991, studies show that 91 percent of people diagnosed with celiac disease had diarrhea. Since 2001, this has dropped to 37 percent! So many doctors are looking for symptoms that the patients do not have.

Practice. Physicians need to put a diagnostic label on a patient in order to initiate treatment. And once you are diagnosed with a condition, the label tends to stick. Although one patient may be easy to treat and another be a nonresponder, the initial diagnosis may not change.

Also, celiac disease is not usually a topic in many of the educational programs physicians attend. However, it is receiving emphasis in some of the medical schools, but it may take years to bring those changes to practicing physicians. Because there are currently no drugs to treat celiac disease, there are no pharmaceutical industry representatives reminding physicians about its diagnosis and treatment.

> *I know someone who just got diagnosed because her doctor retired!*
> (Anonymous, 39)

What Is the Differential Diagnosis of Celiac Disease?

Patients have multiple complaints. Stories abound of people going to different specialists—for diarrhea, osteoporosis, diabetes, peripheral neuropathies, irritable bowel syndrome, anemia, infertility—that are then labeled and treated. Too often these symptoms and tests offer clinical proof of conditions that are never seen as manifestations of one underlying condition.

There are also some patients with symptoms such as continuing fatigue, muscle aches, headaches, and an irritable bowel who are eventually told, "It's all in your head." When tests for everything else are negative, these patients may begin to believe that it is.

> *I just assumed that once you hit middle age, it's supposed to hurt.* (Cindy, 45)

In short, both patient and doctor may be focused on the wrong disease entity or diagnosis.

What, then, are the conditions that tend to mask or divert a diagnosis of celiac disease? Many share *etiology* (origins/causes) and pathology, but each has important characteristics that are worth understanding. And some conditions may occur in conjunction with celiac disease.

Irritable Bowel Syndrome (IBS)

> *My husband had stomach issues and always thought it was a nervous stomach. He was hospitalized six times throughout college*

*complaining of terrible stomach pain. They told him he had IBS. He
runs a big company and thought it was just the stresses of New
York living.*

*He had a terrible, itchy, horrific rash on his shoulders and el-
bows, ever since I've known him. He went to all the dermatologists and used cortisone creams that helped the inflammation a
little.*

*After our daughter was diagnosed with celiac disease, it took
me five months to convince him to do blood work. My daughter's
pediatrician did them and she said: "Look, they're a little elevated:
50 percent of people with your numbers would have it, 50 percent
would not. Go on with your life, move on." He was so happy!*

*I hounded him and made him see a proper "adult" doctor . . .
who looked at the bloods and said: "Plain as day, this is celiac disease. I never saw a better case on paper." He had an endoscopy
and, P.S., he had it.*

*He went on a gluten-free diet and his stomach issues are gone,
bowel issues gone, itching gone, color back in his face, energy level
doubled. Very quickly.* (Ilyssa, 33)

Typically, IBS is a diagnosis reserved for people who do not have another cause for the symptoms and have no "alarm" symptoms such as
weight loss or blood in the stool. IBS is defined by altered bowel movements (alternating diarrhea and constipation) and abdominal pain and
discomfort that are relieved by having a bowel movement.

Gastroenterologists are taught that irritable bowel syndrome is the
most common diagnosis they will make, and this becomes a self-fulfilling
prophecy. Many people have the symptoms and, because it is so common, do not seek health care for them. It is treated by increasing the fiber in the diet and sometimes with pharmaceuticals. Patients are told to
eat seven-grain bread and whole wheat products in addition to other
high-fiber foods. When their symptoms do not get better, or perhaps
grow worse, they go back to the doctor or see other specialists. Until
someone tests for celiac disease, many physicians will not look for another reason for IBS. It is believed that approximately 5 percent of people diagnosed with IBS have celiac disease. Yet about 36 percent of
patients diagnosed with celiac disease have first had a diagnosis of irritable bowel syndrome!

Inflammatory Bowel Disease (IBD)

Inflammatory bowel disease (IBD) encompasses both ulcerative colitis and Crohn's disease (see below). Somewhat confusingly, the category does not include microscopic colitis even though it is an inflammatory bowel disease. (See Chapter 16.)

The symptoms of IBD are very similar to those of celiac disease, including diarrhea, bloating, abdominal pain, and fatigue. The nature of the intestinal inflammation and resulting malabsorption of nutrients is also similar to that found in celiac disease. Symptoms fluctuate over time, and both genetic and environmental factors are involved in the etiology of the diseases. The two profiles are strikingly similar. To complicate matters, you can also have colitis or Crohn's disease in the setting of celiac disease.

Colitis

Colitis is an inflammation of the colon. It is not uncommon to get different kinds of colitis with celiac disease. The most common association is with microscopic colitis or lymphocytic colitis. (See Chapter 16.) In that, the colon looks normal at colonoscopy, but the biopsy shows inflammation. (The pathologist sees an increase in *lymphocytes,* called *intraepithelial lymphocytosis,* similar to what is seen in the small intestine in celiac disease.)

Ulcerative colitis causes chronic inflammation and ulcers in the mucosal lining of the colon. Its symptoms include bloody diarrhea, mucus, and pain. Dehydration may occur, but malnutrition is unusual. Some people get anemia from blood loss.

Crohn's Disease

While colitis occurs in the colon, Crohn's disease is an inflammatory condition that can occur from the mouth to the anus, but most commonly in the small intestine and/or colon. It is characterized by persistent diarrhea, bleeding, cramping, weight loss, fatigue, and fever. Because of its autoimmune nature, it is often associated with other inflammatory conditions that affect the joints, skin, and eyes.

Since Crohn's can cause villous atrophy in the small intestine, it can mask or confuse the celiac disease diagnosis. Blood tests may show antigliadin antibodies (AGA), but not endomysial antibodies (EMA). (See

Blood Tests, Chapter 4.) And celiac disease and Crohn's disease can coexist—thus complicating the diagnosis.

Tropical Sprue

Tropical sprue is a diarrheal illness found in people traveling from or residing in tropical countries. It is thought to be a bacterial infection and is associated with a vitamin B_{12} or folate deficiency. The biopsy can look like celiac disease, but the villous atrophy is patchier in appearance. However, patients do not have positive endomysial antibodies, and it is not related to celiac disease. In fact, it is a variant of bacterial overgrowth.

In the United States, celiac disease is often called nontropical sprue.

Constipation

Patients with constipation who have no complicating factors are usually told to increase their dietary fiber and take a stool softener or over-the-counter laxatives. This is one symptom that most doctors do not equate with celiac disease. The actual mechanism(s) of constipation in celiac disease are not fully understood but may be related to a motility problem in the digestive tract. The constipation often improves on a gluten-free diet, and patients report that the symptoms return if they inadvertently ingest gluten.

Chronic Fatigue

I felt like I was sinking, sinking, sinking into this deep sleep. Like going into a tunnel. (Mary, 50)

Fatigue characterizes illness in general. Infections, blood loss, malabsorption, inflammation, depression—it is the omnipresent symptom. People who are chronically ill are usually chronically tired. Fatigue also characterizes life in the stressful world of the twenty-first century. So its cause(s) can be physical, psychological, or a combination of the two. When other diagnoses have been ruled out, it may be labeled chronic fatigue syndrome, which has been a recognized disease entity since the late 1980s.

Because of the psychological aspects of fatigue, many patients are told it is all in their heads. The difference between the fatigue caused by illness and inflammation and that caused by overwork, physical exertion, or depression is hard to differentiate or diagnose. It is a symptom/

condition much like depression or pain where research is still seeking comparable parameters to determine its source and measure its intensity and effects. Until then, fatigue will most often remain the symptom indicating every disease in the book, or none of them.

Obesity

Obese patients do not get diagnosed with celiac disease because the textbooks say that celiac disease is a malabsorption, wasting syndrome. They get another diagnostic label. But people can be overweight and have celiac disease.

In a study done by the Mayo Clinic in 2003, approximately 20 percent of patients diagnosed with celiac disease were overweight; many were obese, effectively eliminating the definition of celiac disease as a "wasting disease." As described in Chapter 1, the body is extremely efficient at absorbing nutrients. People can have celiac disease in the proximal small intestine and still have many feet of normally functioning intestine to absorb the fats and sugars being eaten. Celiac disease does not discriminate against the overweight or obese and should be considered regardless of the weight of the patient.

Drugs That Mimic Celiac Disease

Olmesartan

We treated a patient at the Center for diarrhea and dehydration severe enough to cause kidney failure and require dialysis. The symptoms mimicked an acute and critical form of celiac disease but were, in fact, caused by Benicar (olmesartan), a drug given to lower blood pressure. It is a very popular class of antihypertensive medications.

Olmesartan can cause intestinal problems that appear to be celiac disease. While the GI effects of Benicar are rare, they can create a potentially life-threatening situation that should be investigated in anyone taking the drug. It can cause damage to the villi of the small intestine, diarrhea, malnutrition, dehydration, and weight loss. These symptoms usually improve dramatically once the drug is stopped.

Immunosuppressants

Also called antirejection drugs, immunosuppressants reduce the strength of the body's immune system, which results in an increased risk of infection and malignancy. All patients receiving an organ transplant take these drugs so that the body will not attack the new organ as "foreign" and reject it.

They are also used to suppress the immune system in autoimmune diseases such as lupus or rheumatoid arthritis, or in severe cases of refractory or unresponsive celiac disease and other inflammatory bowel diseases (e.g., Crohn's, ulcerative colitis) to control intestinal inflammation.

Immunosuppressants are classified into four basic categories that include azathioprine (Imuran), cyclosporine, monoclonal antibodies, and corticosteroids (prednisone). And, while they can stop the crippling effect of many autoimmune diseases, immunosuppressants can also cause injury in the upper GI tract that mimic celiac disease.

Nonsteroidal Anti-Inflammatories

Nonsteroidal anti-inflammatory drugs (NSAIDs) are the main over-the-counter treatment for aches and pains. This grouping includes aspirin, ibuprofen (Advil, Motrin, Nuprin), and naproxen (Aleve). They are also prescribed in stronger form by doctors when needed for more acute pain. Many people take "an aspirin a day" to guard against blood clots. For others with arthritis and sports injuries, NSAIDs are part of their daily regimen.

The most common side effects of NSAIDs are GI problems. Since aspirin is absorbed directly into the bloodstream from the stomach, it does most of its damage there. Some aspirin tablets are available enteric coated so that they are carried further down the GI tract, where they are absorbed and supposedly do less damage. But this can cause changes in intestinal permeability. So, while aspirin saves lives by reducing cardiac events, it can be toxic to the epithelial lining of the gut.

NSAIDs should not be used regularly unless under the guidance of a physician.

Opiates

Opiates are prescription painkillers derived from opium. They slow down the motility (movement) of the GI tract. This can cause delays down the entire length of the gut and constipation. It can also result in nausea, a feeling of fullness after even a small meal, and bloating.

You Think You Are Sick, the Doctor Does Not

I knew there was something the matter with me, but no one would listen—that was stressful and frustrating in itself. I guess I'm living proof the body can learn to live with anything.

I went to twelve gastroenterologists—four tell me it's all in my head. One told me: You're a thirty-nine-year-old female, you're divorced, you own a home, you have to go back to work, sounds to me like you're looking for a husband. How many laxatives do you take a day to give yourself diarrhea? What do you do to make yourself purge? He said I was anorexic. I got up and said: "I'm not going to take this."

I finally saw a gastroenterological specialist and said: "You have to do something." Well, he did a colonoscopy and an endoscopy. The endoscopy came back and he said: "You have celiac disease."
(Anna, 40)

Doctors learn that complaints are not always an indication of an underlying disease. And symptoms do not always correlate to what the doctor finds. The treatment of ulcers is a good example of the conundrum. Endoscopic studies conducted in the early phases of the use of both Tagamet (cimetidine) and Zantac (ranitidine hydrochloride) showed the ulcer had healed, but the symptoms persisted. In some patients, ulcers appeared and there were no symptoms, i.e., the symptoms did not bear any relationship to whether the ulcer was there or not.

Nevertheless, doctors must associate symptoms with test results to make a diagnosis. If they are unable to objectively correlate test results to symptoms, it is more difficult to treat the problem. It is for this reason—because symptoms do not always correlate to what the doctor sees—that the Activity Index was developed.

The Activity Index is a combination of complaints, symptoms, and blood test abnormalities that enables the doctors to "score" patients and determine proper therapy. Patients are treated and doctors assess whether their scores have improved (i.e., gone down). Scoring is used in IBD and Crohn's disease to assess therapies.

Ultimately, celiac disease may not be diagnosed because even though the patients are complaining, the doctors do not take much notice. The doctors end up treating the test data, not the patients.

All told I went to twenty-three physicians before they found out what was wrong with me. I even asked a friend who is a vet. She was the one who said: "Maybe it's a food allergy." (Alice)

Finding a Doctor

Patients complain that it is difficult to find a doctor who is knowledge-able about celiac disease in parts of the United States. We recommend calling the nearest major celiac disease centers or national support groups for a referral. While most gastroenterologists can diagnose celiac disease, few have experience educating patients with persistent symptoms. We also recommend that patients with celiac disease see a registered dietician after diagnosis as following the diet can be difficult.

There are things that make me angry ... misinformation among the major support groups, the price of gluten-free food ... but, most of all, the lack of awareness of celiac disease among the medical profession. It's the most frustrating thing. (Hecky, 43)

Finding the Right Umbrella

Throughout this book are dramatic stories of patients trying to obtain a diagnosis. Many patients simply collect doctors and diagnoses. Each illness has its own textbook. It may take years of unnecessary suffering before the association with celiac disease is found.

So while celiac disease is becoming more well known in the medical and professional communities, it is important for patients to recognize the variable nature of the condition and seek answers for persistent symptoms that defy the diagnostic labels they have been given.

6

Why Do People Get Celiac Disease?

Neither domestic cereals nor milk from hoofed animals is "natural" food in an evolutionary or physiological sense. . . . If there is a single complex of events responsible for the deterioration of human health and ecology, agricultural civilization is it.

—*Paul Shepard*, Coming Home to the Pleistocene

There is no simple answer to why people develop celiac disease. The key mechanisms of the disease involve a complex interaction of genetic and environmental factors—some understood, others not. And the significant initiating factors may change over the course of a person's lifetime and trigger responses that vary in intensity and importance.

Nevertheless, it is interesting and revealing to go back in time in order to understand where celiac disease sprouted.

A Brief History

The crucial transformation—for people with celiac disease—of mankind from hunter/gatherer to agrarian cultivator took place in the eastern Mediterranean and Near East in what is commonly referred to as the Fertile Crescent. It occurred between twelve and eight thousand years ago as mankind began to domesticate plants such as wheat and barley, and animals such as goats, cattle, and sheep. Mankind and wild animals evolved over millions of years: from an evolutionary perspective, the plants and domesticated animals that currently inhabit our lives arrived only yesterday.

As mankind moved from hunter/gatherer to agrarian or pastoralist, intriguing changes occurred in the food supply. We eventually stopped roaming in search of food and began to cultivate and breed what was needed to survive. Domesticated crops and animals were selected and specifically bred for their edibility and usefulness—extra milk, more wool, more meat, larger and more edible grains. The wilderness was pushed farther away, and plants and animals shared the homes, fields, and lives of the agrarian communities.

We selected and cultivated grains and crops that provided nutrition and could be stored for later use, some of which we were not actually designed to digest. Up until then, milk had been available and consumed only during infancy, as it is for all mammals apart from man. But now milk products from domesticated animals were consumed through adulthood and their digestion required the presence of the enzyme lactase. Wheat grains, almost inedible in their wild form, were cultivated to yield the large protein portion that is both nutritious and desirable for making bread, but that contains a complex gliadin amino acid chain that is poorly digested by mankind. Thus the "collision" between gluten and mankind began.

Our ancestors suffered diverse stomach complaints recorded from the early days of written history. No doubt then, as today, this was due to a variety of causes such as infections, disease states, and food intolerances. Whether out of availability, ignorance, or need, we continued to eat food that did not agree with all of us.

"Medicine" as it existed then may not have understood the pathology of indigestion, but the effects of and attempts at cures were also well documented. The Greeks, Romans, and ancient Egyptians wore medical amulets to ward off and/or cure many conditions. Some of the most common involved digestive disorders. Shakespeare immortalized Sir Toby Belch, a literary version of a common problem. The literature about celiac disease took longer to evolve.

The dietary key to the "coeliac"* condition was first described by Samuel Gee in 1888. His contribution was the crucial understanding

---

* *Coeliac* is an alternative spelling for *celiac* usually found outside of the United States.

that "if the patient can be cured at all, it must be by means of diet." At this point in history, celiac disease was life-threatening.

It was not until the 1940s that the diet became more specific. A Dutch physician, Willem Karel Dicke, pointed a finger at "certain types of flour, especially wheat and rye flours." Dicke gained insight into the role of wheat prior to World War II. The deterioration of children with celiac disease in Holland after World War II when bread was reintroduced into their diets confirmed his theories. (He ordered mussels and tulip bulbs as treatment.) Barley was soon understood to be part of the problematic mix. Celiac disease went from life-threatening to treatable.

In the 1950s to 1960s technology progressed to the point that the intestinal biopsy became routine and doctors were able to take samples of the damaged intestine. The initial biopsy instruments were narrow tubes that were passed through the mouth and positioned via X-rays in the upper small intestine. The most commonly used instruments were the Crosby capsule and the Rubin tube. When in position, they were "fired" using suction, removing a large piece of tissue from the jejunum. Hence, the term *suction biopsy*. These instruments were used throughout the world.

During this time, however, a peculiar phenomenon was taking place in the United States. Pediatricians were diagnosing celiac disease without a biopsy. Many children got a diagnostic label of celiac disease or celiac syndrome—some correctly, many not. Pediatricians often used exclusion diets to treat the condition, and most children got better. Many showed no further symptoms when they resumed a normal diet. It is possible that many of these children manifested the disease, in more complex forms, much later in life and that they make up a large percentage of the celiac iceberg that is being uncovered in the United States today.

I was diagnosed the first time as a child, when I was three. I was told I would outgrow it. (Ceil, 43)

I was a celiac baby . . . a banana baby. They told my mother, no lactose, no butter fat, no dairy products. By the time I was eight or nine, I was fine—tall and skinny and pale. All through my teens, I was constantly anemic. Doctors always said in way of explanation: "Ah, you're fair-haired, ah, you're a redhead."

No one ever looked beyond and many still don't today.
(Elaine, 55)

In the 1970s, technology improved again with the development of upper gastrointestinal endoscopy. Doctors could now actually visualize the lining of the intestine. This new procedure was used to obtain biopsy samples of the duodenal mucosa, and tiny (about a millimeter in diameter) pieces of tissue showed pathologic changes just as well as the larger pieces of tissue obtained by the suction biopsy.

As endoscopy and biopsy use became widespread, it was clear that other conditions, apart from celiac disease, could cause similar pathologic changes. As a result, in 1969 a group of well-respected leaders in the field of pediatric gastroenterology, under the auspices of the European Society of Pediatric Gastroenterology, Hepatology, and Nutrition, developed the three biopsy routines for the diagnosis of celiac disease.

The first biopsy was used to demonstrate the abnormalities consistent with the disease; the second, to demonstrate that the pathology would improve with therapy of a gluten-free diet; and the third, to demonstrate that the biopsy would relapse when the child was reexposed to gluten.

This was actually very good medicine! It ensured that the diagnosis of celiac disease was well established before a child was placed on an inconvenient diet that needed to be maintained throughout his or her life. It also ruled out other conditions with similar symptoms and/or an improvement on the diet due to another cause.

By the 1990s, it was clear that, after the age of two years, there were not many other conditions that caused the pathologic appearance of villous atrophy. So, the same group of physicians met and revised the criteria for diagnosis. The revised criteria called for one abnormal biopsy showing villous atrophy for diagnosis and clinical improvement on a gluten-free diet. These criteria have since been applied to adults and are currently the diagnostic standard. (See Endoscopy and Biopsy [the Gold Standard for Diagnosis], Chapter 4.)

The Crucial Pieces of the Puzzle

Why, then, do only certain people have celiac disease and not everyone? The answer is a jigsaw puzzle that is missing some pieces. We know that the development of the disease involves a mixture of genetics and environment, but the total picture is still incomplete.

Gluten

You have to be ingesting gluten to manifest celiac disease; it is the crucial trigger. In fact, celiac disease is the only autoimmune condition in which an environmental trigger has actually been pinpointed. In most other autoimmune diseases, the bodily target for the immune response is understood (the pancreas in diabetes, the myelin sheath in multiple sclerosis, the mucous glands in Sjögren's syndrome), but one environmental villain has not been identified.

None of us digest gluten completely. Some of the peptide chains of gluten—the protein part of wheat that gives bread and cakes the quality we seek—remain intact against the onslaught of intestinal enzymes. It is this fragment of amino acids that appears to set off the immune response that results in celiac disease.

It has been postulated that the response to gluten is both time-related and dose-dependent, but the amount you must ingest to manifest celiac disease and how often has not been determined. The amount of gluten given to children, and the timing of gluten introduction, have both been explored in order to more fully understand the mechanisms of the disease.

Genes

You need to have specific genes in order to develop celiac disease. This is known because 70 percent of identical twins (once one is diagnosed) have the disease and 10 percent of first-degree relatives will have celiac disease. If two siblings are diagnosed, that potential *doubles* for other first- and second-degree members of the family. While some of the specific genes have been identified, it is believed that a number of other genes, as yet to be defined, are also involved, perhaps pivotally.

A Genetic Primer—Fitting the Groove

The key to the celiac puzzle appears to lie in the reaction of specific "sentries" all humans have in their bodies with the undigested gliadin fragment. Human leukocyte antigens (HLA) are proteins found on the surface of almost every cell in the body. They are particularly numerous on white blood cells such as lymphocytes, the immune cells.

HLA antigens patrol the immune system and identify other cells as "self"—belonging to the body—or "nonself"—a foreign substance. They are found on inflammatory cells throughout the lining of the intestine as part of its constant surveillance or inflammatory system. (See What Goes Wrong: The Role of Inflammation, Chapter 2.)

Everyone has a slightly different version of these proteins. Each of us has two sets, one inherited from each parent, and, therefore, each of us reacts differently to different foreign substances. When organ banks are looking for suitable transplant donors or recipients, it is actually the HLA antigens that are used to determine transplant compatibility. This explains the likely match of immediate family members for an organ transplant.

HLA antigens are also thought to play a role in the development of certain genetically predisposed diseases such as diabetes and celiac disease. This is because the genes that predispose people to autoimmune diseases may also control human leukocyte antigens.

The two specific genes that have been recognized so far in celiac disease are part of the HLA class II DQ genes. These genes encode particular HLA proteins that are found on the cell surface, namely HLA-DQ2 and HLA-DQ8.* Ninety-five percent of patients with celiac disease have HLA-DQ2, and most of the remaining 5 percent have HLA-DQ8. The HLA-DQ2, -DQ8 proteins on the surface of lymphocytes are shaped with a groove or furrow that interacts with and binds to the gliadin fragment. In simple terms, specific genetically driven immune cells (lymphocytes with HLA sentries) are primed to react to gliadin.

Friendly Fire

And now, the long gliadin chain that the intestine is unable to digest arrives. As described in Chapter 2, the gliadin chains have been altered by the enzyme tissue transglutaminase (tTG). The chains have been changed into a charged protein with a specific shape that fits into the groove on the surface of the HLA-DQ2 and -DQ8 molecule, which is itself sitting on the surface of lymphocytes in the intestines.

Put simply, after being altered by an enzyme (tTG), gliadin is able to bind more effectively with proteins in the immune system that recognize and protect the body from foreign substances. In some genetically

---

* HLA-DQ2 and -DQ8 are nicknames for genes. They are actually molecules on cells that are encoded by specific alleles of genes: HLA-DQ2 is encoded by alleles DQA1*05, and DQB1*02 and -DQ8 is encoded by DQB1*0302 and DQA1*03.

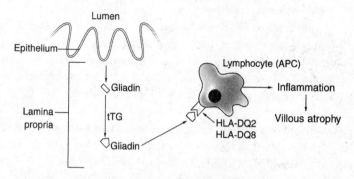

Figure 10. How Gliadin Triggers Villous Atrophy
(APC = Antigen Presenting Cell)

predisposed individuals, this activates an immune response that begins to destroy the cells in the vicinity. The immune cells inappropriately recognize and end up destroying what they were designed to protect. It is an intestinal equivalent of friendly fire.

Therefore, in order to get celiac disease, you have to have gliadin and you have to have HLA-DQ2, -DQ8. Simple enough, but 30 percent of the general population have HLA-DQ2, -DQ8 lymphocytes, while only about 1 percent get celiac disease. And, since 70 percent (not 100 percent) of identical twins and a large percentage in a given family do not have celiac disease, there are obviously other factors at play. And, we now know that there are forty other genes that appear to be important. So it is not clear what genetic influence there is in any one individual except for the absolute necessity to have one of the HLA genes. Therefore, genetics are essential and predisposing, but not determining factors. The answer is not just gluten and genes.

Environment and Genes

Some of the more prominent "other" factors include breast-feeding, infections, pregnancy, and smoking.

Breast-feeding. There is a great deal of evidence that breast-feeding is good for both child and mother. It was formerly believed that fewer breast-fed children develop celiac disease, and when they do, it is at a later age.

However, recent large prospective European studies of children at risk for the development of celiac disease, and a large analysis of all the literature concerning this topic, showed that breast-feeding does not influence the development of the disease. These studies included women that had celiac disease. And, the risk to the child is not influenced by the mother eating, or not eating, gluten while breast-feeding.

Infections. It is clear how the gliadin proteins pass through the intestinal barrier that is designed to keep all foreign bodies out. It is believed that repeated infections, particularly in infancy (and childhood), may play a role. When the lining of the intestine is disrupted by an infection, some larger molecules (such as gliadin) can pass through the tight junctions between epithelial cells and set off the immune reaction.

The small intestine responds to drug therapy and infections—any of which may damage the intestinal lining, making it more permeable and more susceptible to food antigens. Patients diagnosed later in life often see an increase of symptoms, or activation of the disease, after a prolonged or traumatic illness or accident. Similarly, it is often activated after childbirth when the hormonal balance of the body changes. It is unclear whether these events precipitate the onset of symptoms or the disease itself.

Pregnancy. Pregnancy may precipitate symptomatic celiac disease and lead to diagnosis. While the exact mechanism is unclear, pregnancy is a big stress on the body, causes marked hormonal changes, and requires the mother to provide nutrition for the growing child. It is a very well-documented mode of presentation.

Smoking. Several scientific papers have demonstrated that smoking seems to confer some protection against the onset of celiac disease—but its role is very controversial. The mechanisms are unclear. Surprisingly, there is evidence that smoking also protects against ulcerative colitis—nicotine patches are used as therapy for some patients. Conversely, it is known that smoking is a risk factor for Crohn's disease.

Overall, smoking is not healthy for an individual. But in the search to pinpoint the factors that contribute to a tendency to develop celiac disease, any piece of scientific data may be the crucial piece that unlocks the mystery of why one individual with identical genes, eating the same amount of gluten, gets the disease while another does not.

The Microbiome. The intestinal tract is home to trillions of tiny organisms that affect our overall health. These are the bacteria, viruses, fungi, and yeast that compose the microbiota. They line all the surfaces of the body, but most of them exist and flourish in the gut, where they are affected by everything we put in our mouths.

Microbiota are integral to digestion. They release nutrients from foods that would be otherwise indigestible; they make B vitamins and vitamin K; they create a constant state of inflammation and immune regulation to help the body discern friendly from harmful proteins entering the gut. Our microbiota also conduct a constant internal dialogue between the immune, metabolic, and nervous systems.

The different organisms that make up the microbiota are often referred to as commensal bacteria. This derives from the Latin *com* ("in association") and *mansal* ("at the table or meal"). We quite literally "eat at the same table" with our internal microbiotic family. The food we eat is their main source of energy and everything we ingest plays a role in deciding which will thrive and which will perish.

For this reason, microbiota varies not only from individual to individual but in each of us over time. It also differs from country to country depending on what you eat and where you live and is altered when you are sick. Microbiota is an ever-evolving, dynamic, and complex ecosystem.

Diet can alter the composition of your flora and fauna. People on a vegan or vegetarian or very restricted diet can change the composition of their fecal microbiota. Yet the effect of this alteration and whether it returns to a person's "normal" once the diet changes is unclear.

While there is no one "healthy" microbiome, twenty-first-century life, drugs, and changing diets have altered our intestinal ecosystem. Does the disturbance of normal healthy bacteria by antibiotics, acid suppression, and/or age rearrange our intestinal flora or impact our immune systems? Does that impact give certain conditions a chance to flourish or occur? Sometimes "good" bacteria is killed off by antibiotics or other drugs and "bad" bacteria overruns the system, creating disruptions in the microbiota.

Scientists are beginning to explore the possibility that an imbalance of our intestinal microbiota could be another environmental factor contributing to the development of celiac disease as well as other disorders ranging from food allergies and diabetes to obesity. In people whose microbiota respond inappropriately to what is going through the digestive tract, the normal low-grade inflammation that keeps us safe from pathogens goes into overdrive and starts to damage and/or destroy the mucosal lining. There may be a similar genetic/microbiotic/environmental storm at work in celiac disease.

It is important to keep in mind that the microbiome is extremely diverse, even in healthy people, and most diseases have various subtypes and manifestations. Therefore, trying to pinpoint a direct cause-and-effect relation between the microbiome and specific diseases is very difficult. This complex and unpredictable system thrives because of its ability to respond so rapidly to change. First, we need to decode the dialogue between the microbiome and the immune system of the body before we can understand its messages.

A great deal of research is currently underway to determine if manipulation of the microbiota can be used as treatment for infections and illnesses such as celiac disease (i.e., bugs as drugs; see Chapter 27). Changing your diet or taking probiotics or prebiotics in an attempt to alter the microbiome has both short- and long-term effects and is the focus of most of the current research. It is a new frontier in GI health.

The Swedish Epidemic

Scientists were able to explore the interplay of environmental factors in great detail when a population study in Sweden revealed a threefold increase in the occurrence of celiac disease among infants from the mid-1980s to the mid-1990s. This epidemic of celiac disease in children less than two years of age was not occurring in any of the neighboring countries. Examining the years between 1973 and 1997, researchers observed a relationship between both the rise and fall of the epidemic and infant feeding habits.

These observations resulted in a change in advice for breast-feeding and gluten introduction for many countries in Europe. These guidelines advised starting gluten while breast-feeding between four to six months of age.

Subsequent double-blind studies did NOT duplicate these observations and showed that the timing of gluten introduction and breast-feeding within the first twelve months did NOT appear to be determining factors and affect the onset of celiac disease. The amount of gluten ingested was not examined. However, another recent study suggests that the AMOUNT of gluten eaten by babies after twelve months may be an important factor. This highlights the necessity to do controlled scientific studies to duplicate observational findings and determine what is actually occurring.

Infections in the Swedish Epidemic

In the study, there also seemed to be a link to infections that are discussed in terms of a disruption of the barrier function of the small intestine. The Swedish data showed a higher risk for celiac disease in infants who had infections, as well as those born during the summer as compared with winter. This raises interesting questions as to whether the mothers may have had infections in the winter while they were pregnant, or whether the children got more infections during the winter following their birth. It is well known that infections occur more commonly in both children and adults during the winter when people are indoors. Rotavirus infection puts children at risk for celiac disease. In addition, troops returning from the Middle East who had bacterial diarrhea due to campylobacter infections appeared to have a greater chance of acquiring celiac disease.

Socioeconomic Conditions

Interestingly, a lower socioeconomic level was identified as a risk factor in the group below two years of age. This illustrates the complex interaction of environmental and genetic factors in the development of the disease.

Gluten Amounts and Timing of Introduction

Several large studies and analyses have recently looked at whether the timing of gluten ingestion and the amounts of gluten eaten in early childhood affect the risk for celiac disease. These studies have mainly addressed the first twelve months.

These are the results:

1. Timing: Two large prospective European studies showed that neither eating very small amounts of gluten given between four and six months NOR delaying gluten introduction till after twelve months protects from the development of celiac disease.

2. An analysis of all available studies suggested that delaying gluten introduction past seven months did increase the risk somewhat.
3. Amount: The above studies did not address the amount of gluten ingested, but recently analysis of the TEDDY* data suggests that the amount of gluten given to children with a genetic risk factor for celiac disease before two years of age may be a risk factor.

Overall, it appears that gluten should be introduced in small amounts at about six months, and maintained after that, being careful to not give large amounts within the first two years.

Celiac disease has many interacting causes, and when, and whether, it develops is more likely determined by the interaction between an individual's genetic makeup and environmental exposures. Notably, the exposures of importance may vary during a life span.

The Hygiene Hypothesis

It would appear that celiac disease is on the rise, and several recent studies have shown that this increase is not simply due to improved detection and diagnosis. In other words, there appears to be a growing *occurrence* of celiac disease. Interestingly, this appears to be part of the larger scientific observation that autoimmune diseases and allergies are also increasingly more common.

Various theories have been suggested to explain this phenomenon. One intriguing theory, the "hygiene hypothesis," was suggested by Dr. David Strachan in 1989. It proposes that an exposure to infections and unhygienic conditions early in life somehow conveys protection against the development of allergies. The theory has evolved and expanded over the years to explore the role of the environment in the response of the immune system and the development of autoimmune diseases.

Let Them Eat Dirt?

Some scientists feel that the current obsession with personal and household hygiene has led to an increase in allergic reactions. While it is well documented that avoiding germs helps prevent the spread of infections, the hygiene hypothesis suggests that we have taken this too far. By avoiding minor threats early in life, some feel that the immune system has no op-

---

* The Environmental Determinants of Diabetes in the Young

portunity to develop fully. And with the advent of antibiotics and vaccinations, the immune system is no longer required to fight germs as actively as it did in the past. This theory was reinforced by the observation that children growing up on farms had fewer allergies than those in cities.

A recent Finnish study compared rates of celiac disease in Karelia, Russia, to an adjacent Finnish town. The populations in both areas were "equally exposed to grain products and share partly the same ancestry (i.e., gene pool), but live in completely different socio-economic environments." It gave the researchers an almost ideal setting to study the interaction of genes and environment on the development of celiac disease.

The results were intriguing. The prevalence of celiac disease in Russia was 1 in 496, while in Finland it was 1 in 107. Because of the similarity of genetic predisposition and the consumption of grain products, the researchers suggested that the prevalence may be "associated with the protective environment characterized by inferior prosperity and standard of hygiene in Karelia."

Too Clean or Not Too Clean

Before people start feeding their children off the floor, it should be stressed that many researchers feel that the hygiene hypothesis is far too simplistic an approach to the cause of celiac disease or any other autoimmune disease. Others would like to see it renamed as the "microbial exposure/deprivation" hypothesis. This would serve to focus attention on the impact of microbes on disease without discouraging good hygiene practices.

There is no doubt that celiac disease evolves from a series of complex interactions that occur throughout a person's lifetime. The hygiene hypothesis poses an intriguing area for further research but should not be considered as a sole determinant. It certainly provides food for thought.

Epigenetics

Another clue to the development and increasing incidence of celiac disease may lie in the field of epigenetics, an exciting area being explored as a possible bridge between early life events and the risk of disease later in life.

Epigenetics is a term coined in 1942 that describes changes in the expression or behavior of a gene caused by environmental factors. These changes do not affect the underlying DNA but exist "over" or "on top of" (Greek *epi*) the inheritable genetic legacy.

The underlying genetic mechanisms are complex and only partially understood. One way to understand some of them is to think of DNA as an instruction manual for every cell in the human body. If something were to change the font of the manual to a foreign language that the cell could not "read," that gene would be silenced. If the manual were edited to include faulty instructions, the cell would alter its behavior accordingly. It is the environmental—nonevolutionary—changes to this "manual" that scientists are trying to decode and understand. These changes do not affect DNA sequence, only its behavior.

It is hypothesized that if the environment can modify gene expression through epigenetic mechanisms, it may contribute to autoimmune disease in a genetically predisposed person. And genetic damage has been demonstrated in different dietary situations. It is therefore possible that epigenetics may play a role in the recent increase in celiac disease prevalence.

What We Know

We know that celiac disease is a genetic, autoimmune condition that requires exposure to gluten to express itself. It is both common and permanent, although the age of onset ranges from early childhood through late adulthood.

We also know that there are significant gender differences in patients with celiac disease. More women have autoimmune diseases (3:1) than men, and this ratio seems to apply to the incidence of celiac disease as well. But despite the fact that celiac disease is a female-predominant disease, men appear to have more severe manifestations. They appear to have greater malabsorption, manifested by worse bone density. They also tend to develop female-predominant diseases—iron deficiency anemia and autoimmune diseases—at the same rate and severity as women.

We Are Not There Yet

While different genetic, environmental, and immunological factors have been identified, there are still many questions to be answered.

The genetic influence is clearly demonstrated by the prevalence in first-degree relatives and concordance among identical twins, but all of the genes involved in the disease have yet to be conclusively identified.

Researchers are looking for other non-HLA genetic factors because the HLA genes are thought to account for less than 50 percent of the genetic influence. It is also possible that these other genes might account for the variable clinical nature of celiac disease.

The peak age of diagnosis in adults is in the fourth and fifth decades. However, factors that influence the age of onset in adults are unknown.

The exact mechanisms of the gliadin/tTG/HLA immune response are being studied to determine how and where in the process it can be blocked or prevented. Many unanswered questions that are being scrutinized in research today may point the way to a cure, vaccine, or "blocker" for the disease. (See Chapter 27.)

What we do know says a great deal about how far we have to go and the need for further research. It would appear that we are still hunting and gathering.

PART II

RELATED CONDITIONS AND COMPLICATIONS

Celiac disease is a multisystem disorder. Patients will gladly attest to their personal list of hematologists, immunologists, rheumatologists, endocrinologists, neurologists, dermatologists, allergists, psychiatrists, internists, and gastroenterologists to prove the point. The small intestine may be the main target of injury, but the damage does not stop there.

The next eight chapters explore the diverse and far-reaching nature of the disease, and the long journey many patients have taken to the right diagnosis.

7

Neurological Manifestations

At night in bed, my left leg kept falling asleep. This went on for a few days, and I thought I must be sleeping wrong, leaning on one side. After a week or so I finally said: "Something's not right."

Now, I'm a type 1 diabetic and under very good control. I didn't think I had any neurological problem, but given the fact that my leg was falling asleep, and knowing that I'm a type 1, the only thing that came to my mind was peripheral neuropathy (numbness and/or tingling due to damaged nerves).

My diabetes doctor said: "You must be sleeping funny; there's no way you have peripheral neuropathy." So I went to the Internet and punched in peripheral neuropathy and up comes a doctor, an expert on peripheral neuropathy here in New York City. I made an appointment; he checked my knees and made me walk on my toes, etc. He said: "I really can't find anything terribly wrong," but he did a number of blood tests.

About two weeks later I get a letter with the results. He suggested a diagnosis of celiac disease. I had never heard of celiac disease before and looked it up and nearly fell off my chair: bread is one of my favorite foods. The doctor referred me for a biopsy at the Celiac Disease Center at Columbia University. The intestinal biopsy was positive, and they put me on a gluten-free diet. Two weeks later, my leg stopped falling asleep.

My diabetologist had never even raised the consideration of celiac disease. It's basically a miracle how I found out about this. I had no intestinal symptoms. (David, 51)

Everyone, at some point in life, will experience a neurological symptom or condition. It may be as simple as a headache or numbness in a limb, or as complex as a seizure, stroke, or paralysis.

The nervous system and the brain are among the most intricate and most elusive parts of the human body. With a reach that extends into and out of every nook and cranny of our being, the nervous system regulates and monitors all of the organs and systems of the body and controls our motor and sensory activities and behavior. It is also intimately involved in our perception of the world and our experience of pain.

Often, neurological conditions are the only manifestations of celiac disease that a patient may experience. For patients like David, they are among the most common symptoms of celiac disease that are considered atypical and delay diagnosis. David was experiencing the manifestations of a peripheral neuropathy, numbness and tingling (paresthesia), which are regularly seen in patients with other diseases such as longstanding diabetes. Without his persistence in defining the underlying cause of his discomfort, and looking beyond the "obvious" diabetic link, his celiac disease would have gone undiagnosed for years.

The well-defined neurological associations with celiac disease include the following:

- Peripheral neuropathies (numbness and/or tingling in the hands and feet)

- Ataxia (a balance disturbance)

- Epileptic seizures, with and without intracranial calcifications (calcium deposits in the brain), particularly in children

- Migraines

- Brain atrophy and dementia (deteriorated mentality)

Any one of these complications may affect as many as 8 to 10 percent of people with celiac disease. But it is important to note that none of these diseases are necessarily related to one another—the parts of the nervous system associated with each of these conditions are totally separate.

The Nervous System 101

The nervous system is composed of two parts:

- The central nervous system (the brain, brain stem, and spinal column)
- The peripheral nervous system (a system of nerve fibers that relay messages to and from the central nervous system to all parts of the body)

Nerve/neuron networks radiate throughout every inch of the body. They are part of a highly complex, balanced system of excitatory and inhibitory mechanisms that control our body functions, systems, and perceptions. A delicate balance, or homeostasis, between these mechanisms is crucial to function.

A good example is balance. Nerve fibers are continually assessing the position of our limbs (through position and touch fibers) and compensating (exciting/inhibiting) for movement in order to keep us upright and in balance. We are not aware of this mechanism unless it goes awry.

The instantaneous reaction we have when we touch a hot stove is another good example. Excited pain fibers in the nerves relay the message up to the brain that the hand has been burned. Motor responses are relayed back that cause us to move the hand away and simultaneously scream "Ouch!" All of these mechanisms are imperceptible and occur in milliseconds in order to enable and protect the body.

It is for good reason that we are all a bundle of nerves.

When the message impulses relayed throughout these systems become blocked or distorted, neurological symptoms occur. A *neuropathy* is the syndrome, sometimes called neuritis, caused by the inflammation of nerves. When nerves get inflamed, they cannot function properly, which may result in altered sensation of pain, touch, or position as well as weakness or balance problems.

Peripheral Neuropathy

Peripheral neuropathy is a general term given to the conditions in which the nerves in the body's extremities (i.e., the peripheries) do not perform properly. This may be the result of:

- Infection
- Trauma
- Inflammation
- Autoimmune factors
- Toxins or poisons

The result is an alteration of normal sensation. Symptoms will correlate with the main grouping of nerves affected. If the sensory nerve fibers are affected, there may be numbness, tingling, pressure or pain, or a lack of perception of pain so that burns or traumatic events may not be perceived. If the sensory nerves that relay information about position or touch are affected, balance problems will result. If motor nerves are affected, weakness can occur.

In a peripheral neuropathy, the most distant parts of the body such as hands, fingers, feet, toes, nose, face, and tongue are affected. The peripheral neuropathy seen in celiac disease is mainly sensory—motor effects (weakness) are seen less frequently. Approximately 10 percent of people who have peripheral neuropathies with no obvious cause actually have celiac disease.

Peripheral neuropathies can be mild (a foot that falls asleep at night, tingling in the fingers) or it can be severe (an inability to hold a toothbrush or pen, the sensation of constant pain that makes it impossible to tolerate normal activities). For patients and doctors alike, the association between these symptoms and a diseased GI tract appears obscure.

Nerve Conduction Studies (EMG)

Nerve conduction studies are used to measure the conduction of nerve impulses in large nerves and assess the extent of damage to them. Peripheral neuropathies may affect the small nerve fibers—not the larger nerves tested in EMG. Therefore, these studies may be normal in people with celiac disease who have a peripheral neuropathy. Patients have altered sensation—a neuropathy—but a normal conduction study. The neurologists conclude that there is nothing wrong because they cannot measure it.

A promising diagnostic tool is being developed in which a skin biopsy is taken in order to examine the small microscopic nerve fibers. The biopsy examines both the density of these small nerve fibers and the presence of inflammation. This test would ascertain the involvement of small microscopic nerves whose function cannot be assessed in the EMG study.

Treatment for peripheral neuropathies is a strict gluten-free diet and pain medications and/or anti-inflammatories. (See The Effect of the Gluten-Free Diet, page 97.)

Ataxia

Ataxia is a balance disturbance caused by a loss of position and motor coordination. Patients complain of unsteadiness, exaggerated movements or overshooting the mark, and falling easily.

In various studies, approximately 9 to 15 percent of patients with ataxia of unknown origin have celiac disease.

Ataxia may be related to diseases affecting different parts of the nervous system, including:

- Changes in the cerebellum (which controls balance)
- Changes in the brain stem (which sends motor messages to the body)
- Changes in the peripheral nerves (we sense where we are because of information coming in from our peripheral nerves; if these nerves are unable to send messages, balance can be affected because the limbs cannot properly perceive where they are)

Ataxia is one of the most frequent neurological syndromes associated with celiac disease and is often seen without any GI complications.

Epilepsy

More than one million Americans have recurrent seizures. Epilepsy is the second most common major neurological disorder after stroke.

In patients with celiac disease, the incidence of epilepsy has been reported to range from 3 to 5 percent.

Epilepsy is caused by an intermittent, spontaneous electrical activity or discharge in the brain. These spontaneous "spikes" disrupt the normal baseline electrical rhythms that we all have whether awake or asleep. They excite the neurons near them, which results in inappropriate activity. If the inappropriate activity is in the part of the cerebral cortex that controls motor activity, abnormal movements, or a convulsion, will result. If the abnormal activity is in the visual cortex, vision may be affected. Similarly, other areas of the senses may be targeted.

Grand mal seizures, or convulsions, involving the whole body can also occur, accompanied by a loss of consciousness.

There are different forms of epilepsy:

- *Grand mal,* which is a generalized seizure
- *Petit mal,* or focal seizures, in which people may experience olfactory or mood changes

There are many reasons for people to have seizures, including trauma, scar formation in the brain, or metabolic problems such as magnesium or calcium imbalances.

The relationship between epilepsy and celiac disease may simply be the occurrence of two relatively common diseases in the same patient. For others, especially in children, the connection is more clearly defined.

Cerebral Calcifications: A Recognition Factor for Celiac Disease

The specific type of epilepsy directly related to celiac disease is a relatively uncommon syndrome of occipital calcification and epilepsy. It has been studied in both pediatric and adult populations, but it appears to be mainly a pediatric syndrome.

Calcium deposits appear in the occipital (rear) part of the brain and are associated with epilepsy. The calcifications were initially thought to be due to folate insufficiency, but they are now believed to be an autoimmune phenomenon. The presence of this syndrome should trigger a consideration of celiac disease. It may improve on a gluten-free diet.

Migraines

> I've suffered from migraines my whole life... maybe two days a month I don't have one. I had CAT scans and all these workups. I'm on Imitrex. After two months on the gluten-free diet, the headaches were cut in half. (Ilyssa, 33)

Migraines are industrial-strength headaches. They occur periodically, come on rapidly, and are caused by the constriction and dilation of the intracranial arteries. A recent study on blood flow abnormalities in the brain showed a direct correlation between untreated celiac disease and blood flow alterations. In this study, 4 percent of migraine patients (versus 0.4 percent in the control group) had celiac disease.

Many patients with celiac disease complain of various degrees of headaches and migraines that improve in both severity and occurrence on a gluten-free diet. (See The Effect of the Gluten-Free Diet, page 97.)

Other Neurological Conditions

There are several reports in the literature of patients with *dementia* who were found to have celiac disease. In Finland, researchers found five patients with celiac disease who developed dementia before the age of sixty. A study from the Mayo Clinic identified thirteen patients with cognitive impairment and personality changes that occurred with the development of celiac disease.

While one recent study on Alzheimer's failed to show a clear association, other cognitive studies are needed to assess the relationship between mental status and cognitive function and celiac disease or non-celiac gluten sensitivity.

Paralysis

We were on a vacation in Puerto Rico and Lily got really sick. She was eleven months old and we gave her bananas and rice and all the things you're supposed to give for diarrhea, and she kept getting progressively worse. So, we go home and go to our own doctor, who said, "Just give her the rice and bananas and tea diet."

Lily was a nine-pound, eight-ounce baby—she was born big. During her one-year checkup, she was seventeen or eighteen pounds. She had not yet doubled her weight at one year of age. I remember being concerned, but the doctor just said: "She must be the runt in the family; she's just small, don't worry."

A week or two after she turned one, she had a rash all over her body and a high fever for twenty-four hours, and then it went away. During the high fever, I brought her to her pediatrician and he gave the rash some crazy name and said: "Just take her home, she'll be fine." By the following week, she wasn't waving hello and goodbye anymore, or holding on to the coffee table and cruising around. We were trying to get her to stand on her own and she couldn't; her legs just gave out. I was carrying this baby all over the place.

When I look back at her one-year pictures with her party dress on and tiara, she looks like a cancer patient. Her hair was barely there. Her eyes were sunken. Her belly was sticking out. Her legs were like nothing. But nobody saw anything. The pediatrician never saw anything, and we were thinking this is what she always looked like. This is who Lily is.

I took her back to the doctor and said: "What's going on?" He said: "Don't worry, she's tired from the virus; sometimes it takes time to get your energy level back." That made sense. But two days later she wasn't doing anything. She wasn't walking, cruising, just lying there. She was losing all her milestones and just looked as if she was getting worse.

So I called the doctor and said: "I need an orthopedist—this baby can't walk anymore." He said, "You need a neurologist"... who took one look and said: "There is something very wrong with her." They thought she might have a tumor on her spine, which is why she wasn't going to be able to walk anymore.... My husband and I are discussing moving to a house with one floor because she's going to have to be in a wheelchair....

So they send her to the PICU (pediatric intensive care unit). They do a spinal tap, comes back fine. Then she gets an MRI—I'm singing to her outside of that crazy machine for an hour—and that's totally fine. After four days of testing—I've never cried so much in my life watching what they were doing to her—she came home with a diagnosis of postviral syndrome. She's down to sixteen pounds, losing weight rapidly, and now she really looks like she's dying....

Then the doctor calls and says: "Your daughter has celiac disease. She cannot eat gluten." I had never heard of the word gluten before. I thought, "How am I feeding this child?" At first it was just bananas, rice, vegetables, potatoes, and meat... pure food... nothing else. But ten days after being on that diet, all the kids were upstairs in my room watching TV, and she pulled to stand and they're all screaming: "Mommy, Mommy, Lily's walking!!"

I really feel that the neurologist saved her life. What's the point in tracking your weight? What's the point of all this health care management where you have to go to the pediatrician every three months? She never doubled her weight at a year and nobody saw anything. Not even me, nobody. Just think of all the hundreds of thousands of dollars that the hospital spent; the trauma for all of us being in a hospital for five days and letting it get so far. Think of what could have been prevented if my pediatrician said: "Why don't we just give her a blood test for celiac disease?" (Sue, 41)

Lily had acute paraplegia: she could not use her legs. The neurologist felt this was due to a severe neuropathy. Her symptoms started with a rash, fever, and fatigue, and she soon could not stand. She had become wasted and her abdomen distended without anyone really noticing. Then she lost muscle tone and muscle power. She was admitted to the pediatric intensive care unit where doctors, after reviewing her growth charts, discovered that she had stopped growing after the fifth month. This combined with her general neuropathy suggested to the neurologist that Lily could have celiac disease.

In weeks after starting a gluten-free diet, she could walk again. Essentially, when the cereals came in, the mind and body went out. Lily's story is one about a reversible kind of neurological damage. There is evidence that the earlier the diet is started, the more likely it is that the damage can be reversed.

What Causes Neuropathies in Celiac Disease?

There are many underlying causes of neuropathies that include physical trauma to the nervous system, damage to the vascular supply to the nerves because of underlying illness or trauma, diseases that affect any part of the nervous system (stroke, multiple sclerosis, etc.), vitamin deficiencies, inflammation, or autoimmune factors.

The neuropathies commonly found in celiac disease appear to be related to the three latter factors.

Vitamin Deficiency

When patients go to a doctor with a neurological complaint, the physician must rule out vitamin or mineral disturbances/deficiencies:

- Low calcium or magnesium can cause convulsions and paresthesias.
- A vitamin B_{12} deficiency can cause peripheral neuropathy, balance disturbances, and dementia.

- A vitamin E deficiency can cause sensory loss or ataxia.
- Excess vitamin B$_6$ can cause a painful neuropathy.

If vitamin or mineral deficiency is the problem, the condition re-solves itself with vitamin or mineral supplements; excess is resolved by stopping the medication.

Most of the cases of neurological problems in celiac disease are not as easily remedied because they most often occur in the absence of vita-min deficiencies. But, given the malabsorption problems of many pa-tients, this is an obvious cause that must be investigated.

Inflammation

Inflammation may occur as part of the autoimmune reaction, and that is considered to be the main mechanism of the inflammatory response in celiac disease.

Inflammation levels can be measured through serological tests. The two tests that measure inflammation in the body are the *erythrocyte sedi-mentation rate (ESR)* and the *C-reactive protein (CRP)*. The ESR is measured by calculating how fast the red cells (erythrocytes) settle in a test tube. If there are abnormal constituents in the blood, they interfere with the sedi-mentation rate of the cells. Neither the ESR nor the CRP is specific for any condition or organ; the results simply indicate inflammation in the body.

A very high ESR occurs in conditions such as a malignancy, chronic inflammatory conditions, or rheumatoid arthritis. Patients with celiac dis-ease often have a very high ESR. This is not unexpected, since a lot of in-flammation in a very large organ like the intestine (see What Goes Wrong: The Role of Inflammation, Chapter 2) can elevate the sedimentation rate. A recent study demonstrated that the ESR goes down on a gluten-free diet.

Autoimmune Reaction

The autoimmune connection between celiac disease and neuropathies is thought to be due to an antibody against brain tissue, or an antibody to a component of the nerve. An antibody that we have found to be ele-vated in some patients with neuropathy and celiac disease is the anti-ganglioside antibody. This reacts against a component of the nerves.

Some studies suggested that ataxia may be caused by an autoim-mune phenomenon. Antibodies to nerves were found in the parts of the brain responsible for the condition.

Several studies have measured the antibodies found in celiac disease—IgA and IgG antigliadin antibodies (AGA)—in patients with various neurological problems. The studies showed that AGA levels are elevated in people with neurological syndromes of unclear origin. They are *not* elevated in those having syndromes and symptoms with a definable cause. For example, more patients with a peripheral neuropathy for which there is no cause have an elevated AGA than patients with an inherited peripheral neuropathy.

It is therefore possible that gliadin may be a trigger for neurological issues even in the absence of celiac disease.

The Effect of the Gluten-Free Diet

The effect of therapy is difficult to assess in neurological complaints. Different medications, doses, and diets ameliorate symptoms for one patient and not another. The overall response to a gluten-free diet is equally mixed.

Some patients, such as David, report a complete reversal of symptoms on a gluten-free diet. There are other patients with peripheral neuropathies who appear to get symptoms when ingesting gluten and whose symptoms become less severe on the diet. Yet other patients develop peripheral neuropathies while *on* a gluten-free diet.

Because all patients do not appear to respond to the diet, there are other therapies—including drugs such as Neurontin, IV gamma globulin, nonsteroidal anti-inflammatories—that can be employed.

Similarly, there is conflicting data on the effect of the gluten-free diet on ataxia. Some patients show improvement after one year on the diet. Treatment with IV gamma globulin has also produced improvement in some patients.

The control of seizures in people with celiac disease seems to improve or stabilize on a gluten-free diet, particularly if the diagnosis and diet occur soon after the onset of epilepsy. Drug therapy is often needed as well. The incidence of cerebral calcifications and epilepsy has been observed to be lower in celiac disease patients who are following a gluten-free diet.

There are still many areas of the nervous system, as well as its relation to celiac disease, that remain to be revealed. What is clear is that both patients and doctors must excite a neurological connection if the celiac iceberg is to be exposed.

8

Malignancy

Around my first birthday doctors announced that I had celiac/sprue. They put me on a special diet where I ate a certain type of milk and bananas. That was my food. The war was on, and bananas were impossible to get. About five or six years later they pronounced me cured.

Things went along well, seemingly, for fifty-five years. Then I started getting stomachaches. I also had cramps in my legs. When our friends started telling my wife I really didn't look so good, that I looked pale, she made me go to the doctor.

The doctor thought I might have a vitamin K deficiency and did some blood tests. The results came back that I was anemic. I went into the hospital for an endoscopy and they found a cancer (adenocarcinoma) of the small intestine. It was stage 3: it had spread to some lymph nodes. The doctor said it was from years of neglect from the celiac disease. He had to leave something (a microscopic cancer growth) in a touchy area and said: "We're going to be hearing from this cancer again." I went on chemo for a year.

A few years later the microscopic growth had gotten bigger, and they went back in and cut everything out. And I've been fine since then. That was four years ago. It's a matter of luck I'm sitting here talking to you. (Fred, 63)

While it is accurate to say that celiac disease is a multisystem disorder that is associated with many other problems, cancer is one of the major complications of the disease. *Malignancy* is a word that worries both patient and doctor—a diagnosis of cancer will overwhelm the diagnosis of celiac disease. And malignancies occur more commonly in patients with long-standing celiac disease—particularly those who were told they had "outgrown" the condition.

Patients with celiac disease have an increased mortality rate that exceeds that of the general population. This has been shown in many studies from Europe. The increased mortality is believed to be due mainly to the development of non-Hodgkin's lymphoma. The overall risk for malignancy for specific cancers in people with celiac disease has been reported at anywhere from nine to thirty-four times greater than that of the general population.

High-risk malignancies for patients with celiac disease include:

1. *Thyroid cancer.* We have determined that the risk for thyroid cancer appears to be twenty-two times that of the general population.
2. *Adenocarcinoma of the small intestine.* Adenocarcinoma of the small intestine is extremely uncommon in the general population and holds a comparatively high risk for those with celiac disease. And while celiac disease is predominantly female (3:1), most of the reported cases of small intestinal adenocarcinoma were in men.
3. *Lymphoma.* The predominant celiac-disease-associated lymphomas are non-Hodgkin's lymphoma of any type: T cell, B cell, and mantle cell. Also, they can occur not only in the intestine but at any site, including the skin, brain, or lymph nodes throughout the body. The most well-known associated lymphoma is the rare enteropathy-associated T-cell lymphoma (EATL). It is typically poorly responsive to chemotherapy.

   Recent studies show the risk of people with celiac disease developing non-Hodgkin's lymphoma to be seven to nine times that of the general population. This is still a significant risk, but not as high as previously reported.
4. *Esophageal cancer—mainly squamous.* Head and neck squamous cancers occur more commonly in patients with celiac disease. This includes squamous carcinomas of the tongue, mouth, tonsils, and pharynx, as well as of the esophagus. Squamous cell cancers of the skin are not increased in celiac disease.
5. *Melanoma.* The significantly increased risk of melanoma seen in our study may be due to the recognition of a persistent increase in

the incidence of melanoma in the United States. This has started to slow in recent years.

6. *Malignancy in childhood.* A recent study suggested that malignancy in childhood celiac disease is underreported. A study by the European Society of Gastroenterology, Hepatology, and Nutrition uncovered twenty-one new cases of cancer in children with celiac disease. More research is needed to determine whether celiac disease is a risk factor for the development of malignancies in childhood.

Celiac disease appears to be protective against the development of breast cancer. The mechanism of this is unclear.

The Relationship of Malignancies and Celiac Disease: What Is the Risk?

1. *Long-standing celiac disease.* The greatest risk for malignancy is before a patient is diagnosed, especially if the patient has long-standing celiac disease.

2. *Believing that you have "outgrown the disease."* Many children and adults with celiac disease go on a gluten-free diet, resolve their symptoms, and then ingest gluten and feel no ill effects. In reality, the only things they have "grown out of" are the symptoms! **Celiac disease is a lifelong illness.**

In the United States, pediatricians regularly use exclusion diets for children with GI complaints. This may in fact be treating some children for celiac disease—unknowingly and without a diagnosis. Children feel well on a gluten-free diet—and eventually feel equally well when they do eat gluten. So everyone thinks that the problem has disappeared. But this early treatment without diagnosis may result in a more sinister form of occult celiac disease. The patient feels well and is at risk for a complication developing later in life, such as adenocarcinoma of the small intestine.

3. *Not adhering to a gluten-free diet.* Gluten is the environmental trigger that initiates the damage to the gut and, in turn, the body. It must be removed to halt the destructive process. Although there is little research into the long-term effects of small amounts of gluten in the diet, it is generally believed that even small amounts may

continue to trigger undesirable outcomes. The continuing ingestion of gluten—i.e., noncompliance to the diet, either intentional or unintentional—is the major risk factor for malignancy.

Many patients with dermatitis herpetiformis (the itchy, blistering skin manifestation of celiac disease) are put on drugs to repress their symptoms and then continue to eat gluten. These patients are at a higher risk of developing a lymphoma, similar to the risk in those with celiac disease.

What Causes the Cancers?

The mechanism(s) underlying the development of different cancers are not completely understood. This is equally true for the development of malignancies in patients with celiac disease. Our studies have shown that the major factor associated with the development of lymphoma is failure to heal the gut. It is a good argument for having a repeat biopsy to document healing. Several other factors are being studied:

- *Increased intestinal permeability.* A "leaky gut," or the increase in intestinal permeability that accompanies celiac disease, may allow patients with celiac disease to absorb toxins and carcinogens more readily than those without celiac disease.
- *The inflammatory process.* Chronic inflammation and inflammatory stimulation (see Chapter 2) are believed to play a role in many of the self-destructive mechanisms in celiac disease. The body literally attacks itself in autoimmune disease and the cancer mechanism may be involved in, or feed off of, this complex process. Persistent inflammation has long been examined as a risk factor for cancer. This is well known in the field of gastroenterology and is thought to be the mechanism for the development of cancer in patients with chronic ulcerative colitis and Barrett's esophagus. The inflammation results in chronic irritation and tissue turnover/replacement, which increases the cancer risk.
- *Immune surveillance.* The immune system of people with celiac disease is continually turned on or stimulated. Somehow, this allows the normal mechanisms by which we protect ourselves to be overwhelmed. Everyone regularly develops malignant or potentially malignant cells. These cells are detected and "killed" by our immune system. Over time this mechanism becomes less active, causing the

development of cancers as we age. In celiac disease, the mechanism of immune surveillance may be generally less active or overcome.

- *Genes.* Some people may have a genetic tendency for certain cancers. This has been explored in other cancers (e.g., breast and ovarian) but not in the celiac-disease-related malignancies.
- *Nutritional deficiencies.* People who are nutritionally compromised are at an increased risk for a variety of problems. While the specifics are not clearly, scientifically defined, there is the potential for an increase in malignancies.

Specific vitamin deficiencies are associated with malignancy, including the link between vitamin A deficiency and squamous cell cancers such as those associated with the mouth and throat. But, that does not seem to be the mechanism in patients with celiac disease.

Food toxins, sensitivities, allergies, and intolerances have, in one form or another, been blamed for triggering malignant reactions. Specific deficiencies usually receive equal treatment. There are currently no definitive scientific studies linking specific nutritional deficiencies to the cancers found in celiac disease.

Management Issues

Patients on a gluten-free diet who are recovering from a cancer often ask the following questions:

Q: How compliant do I have to be?
A: Very.

Q: What if I get gluten through cross contamination?
A: Learn the diet, control the things you can, and focus on getting better.

Q: What will happen if I eat one slice of pizza?
A: You will rev up your immune system and no one knows the exact results of this. It may make getting better difficult or impossible. If you have one "hit" of gluten—as small as one-eighth teaspoon—you are going to get an inflammatory response and immune reaction that lasts a certain period of time—the half-life of the inflammatory mediators. In other words, the inflammatory response and white cells called into the

area will be active for a period of time and then fade off. With persistent "hits" of gluten, the inflammation and response never fade and the intestine never has time to heal.

The management of malignancies and celiac disease focuses primarily on the cancer in the presence of a strict gluten-free diet.

The Effect of the Gluten-Free Diet

A gluten-free diet is considered protective against the development of malignancy. While there is no evidence that a gluten-free diet will cure an established cancer, persistent gluten ingestion is one of the risk factors and may affect healing.

The risk factor is reduced after three to five years on a gluten-free diet, except in the case of non-Hodgkin's lymphoma. There, the risk persisted in several studies despite the gluten-free diet. In other studies, the diet appeared to be protective against the development of this malignancy as well as the others. This is clearly an area where more long-term research is needed.

Should I Be Screened for Cancers?

There are no published guidelines for screening patients with celiac disease for malignancies. But because of the reported increase in a variety of malignancies involving different organs and parts of the body, it is important for people with celiac disease to remain under good health care. This involves:

- Receiving a regular, good physical exam; palpating and looking for enlarged lymph glands and an enlarged spleen or liver is very important in finding cases of lymphoma
- Blood tests that screen for evidence of bleeding or other anomalies
- Regular mammograms (age appropriate), prostate exams, colonoscopies, and gynecological exams per the usual recommendations

These regular exams should enable physicians to locate those few people who might develop a malignancy. Patients with specific symptoms (e.g., rectal bleeding, night sweats) are often tested repeatedly in order to exclude a malignancy. Both doctor and patient are aware of the potential risk and want to ensure that the patient does not have a malignancy. Statistically, the chances are low for someone with celiac disease to develop a malignancy.

There is a great deal more to be learned about the relationship between celiac disease and the malignancies that occur more commonly in people with the disease. While the mechanisms causing the malignancies are not known, the risks go down after three to five years on the diet. Therefore, they are somehow related to having celiac disease.

It is important that these connections are studied and more clearly defined. Hopefully, the links to malignancies and other complicated diseases are on the research horizon.

The important point is that patients with celiac disease get better once they get a diagnosis and go on the diet, and the risk of getting most malignancies decreases.

9

Osteoporosis

The secret life of belly and bone.

—*Delmore Schwartz*

I was anemic for years. When I went to doctors they would say "You have your period," or "You're in high school/college—you don't eat right." I started seeing a hematologist who put me on iron. But when I took it, it would make me so sick. I had stomach pain. I was constipated. So I went to a gastroenterologist, who told me there was nothing there; it was all related to taking iron. He said to take Metamucil.

I never felt right. I was very tired and was always leaving work to go to a doctor—half a day here, half a day there. That summer (1999), I was out with my sister on a beautiful, cool day, and I was sweating. She asked me if I was going through menopause! (I was twenty-six.) I went to my gynecologist, who did blood work—it came back like a woman in her fifties. She sent me to a reproductive endocrinologist, who did many tests—scans, sonograms, more blood work. My blood calcium levels were off, so she sent me for a bone scan and found out I was osteopenic (a precursor of osteoporosis) and osteoporotic (fragile bones susceptible to fractures)!

At this point I started to get bloating. At night my stomach looked like I was seven or eight months pregnant. I went to another gastroenterologist and he told me I had irritable bowel syndrome. He gave me a drug that helped the upset stomach, but the side effects were awful so I stopped taking it. I started losing weight—around twenty pounds once the GI problems kicked in. My mom kept asking me if I was anorexic.

I saw the hematologist for three years, my gynecologist and a reproductive endocrinologist, two gastroenterologists, and four endocrinologists. No one put it all together.

Finally, when I fell and broke my arm, the orthopedist said: "Unless you're an old woman with osteoporosis, you should never have broken a bone in that place." He gave me the name of my fifth endocrinologist (at the Metabolic Bone Disease Center at Columbia), who looked at all the paperwork from the other doctors and said: "You have celiac disease."

I had an endoscopy to confirm the diagnosis and went on the gluten-free diet. I thought: "I'm going to go on a diet and everything will be okay—I don't have to take medication. This is awesome—I'm finally going to feel better." (Lori, 34)

Osteoporosis, literally "porous bones," is a widespread medical problem that affects ten million people in the United States today.* Eighteen million more have low bone mass, placing them in danger of developing the condition. Osteoporosis costs an estimated $18 billion each year in hospital, rehabilitation, and medical care. For patients with celiac disease, the cost goes well beyond the financial.

Osteoporosis is one of the most common complications of celiac disease. Approximately 75 percent of newly diagnosed patients with celiac disease have some degree of bone loss. Recent studies show that up to 35 percent of adults who are newly diagnosed with celiac disease have *established* osteoporosis. While both osteoporosis and celiac disease are more common in women, low bone density is an equal-opportunity complication in the celiac community. And men with celiac disease tend to have more severe osteoporosis.

Much like celiac disease itself, osteoporosis is a "silent" condition. It may develop for years, or even decades, and announce its presence only when a fall or broken bone reveals the extent of the problem. By then, much of the damage is done, and the restoration of normal bone density is difficult.

---

* National Osteoporosis Foundation

The risk of fracture increases as your bone mineral density decreases. This puts most patients with celiac disease at increased lifetime risk for a broken bone. Nevertheless, the specific studies on fracture rates in the celiac disease community show conflicting data. One study puts the risk at that of the general population with osteoporosis. That is a dire warning: one out of every two women and one out of every eight men over fifty will have an osteoporosis-related fracture in their lifetime.

Lori's story exemplifies the wide array and long duration of symptoms, and the many physicians patients must see before someone "puts it all together." But it is important to note that it is highly unusual for a young person to have osteoporosis. This should raise red flags for both patient and doctor and initiate a search for the underlying cause.

Fortunately, Lori is doing very well on the diet. Her bone density has normalized, the anemia is corrected, and both the fatigue and IBS symptoms have improved. If she had been diagnosed earlier, she might have been able to prevent her multiple medical problems, all of which are manifestations of celiac disease.

Bones 101

Most bone formation and building takes place during childhood, adolescence, and early adulthood. After that, it is all downhill. Bones naturally thin after the mid-twenties and this trend accelerates after menopause in women.

Bone, the Calcium Reservoir

Bone is a living, breathing tissue composed mainly of calcium and phosphate. Calcium is one of the most important and most abundant minerals in the body. The body absorbs the calcium it requires from the food we eat and stores excess in the skeletal reservoir. This reservoir not only supports the body and protects many of our internal organs, but our bones also maintain normal levels of calcium in the bloodstream.

The calcium in our bloodstream is an important part of the bone/celiac disease story. Calcium is indispensable to functions throughout the entire body. It is required for muscle function—including heartbeat—as well as for nerve transmission. And the need to supply calcium for the body takes precedence over the skeletal function of bone, sometimes to its detriment.

Remodeling the Skeleton

Bone is constantly undergoing "remodeling"—being broken down and built up—throughout our lifetime. Remodeling is affected by a variety of factors:

- Physical activity and weight-bearing exercises build bone.
- Growth factors, including the normal sex hormones—testosterone and estrogens—are required for normal bone growth.
- A lack of dietary calcium (or vitamin D; see page 109) causes a drop in blood calcium levels and increases the *breaking down* processes to provide calcium for the bloodstream.
- Excessive levels of various hormones cause bones to be broken down more rapidly. These include steroids and thyroid hormone.
- Inflammation anywhere in the body causes inflammatory mediators or cytokines to circulate in the blood. These act to interfere with bone formation.

When calcium is needed by the body, it calls for it. Hormones act on the intestine so that calcium is absorbed in larger quantities from the food we eat, and it is *resorbed* or taken out of bone.

Problems begin when the intestine is damaged and unable to absorb calcium. And most calcium is absorbed in the upper small intestine, where celiac disease exerts its greatest damage.

The Reservoir Runs Dry

When the necessary supply of dietary calcium is interrupted—through malabsorption or inadequate dietary calcium—the body "borrows" from the bone reservoir and breaks down the bone. Eventually, it runs out of raw materials to rebuild, and the reservoir starts to dry up—the bone becomes brittle and porous and loses calcification.

Bone eventually loses its ability to hold up the weight of the body—producing the "dowager's hump" or stooped-over look of many elderly people with bone deterioration. A fall can cause brittle bones to break more easily.

The three bone disorders seen in patients with celiac disease are osteoporosis, osteopenia, and osteomalacia.

In osteoporosis, the outer shell of the bone becomes thinner and the inner matrix, or core of the bone, loses density. The bone becomes more fragile.

Osteopenia is characterized as a lesser degree of reduction in bone density.

Osteomalacia is characterized by decalcified, *soft* bones. It is usually due to a vitamin D or calcium deficiency and cannot be properly diagnosed without a bone biopsy. Under a microscope, the bones appear only partially formed with an uncalcified matrix. Osteomalacia in a child will cause rickets, or bent bones, characterized by bowed legs. Osteomalacia is rarely diagnosed in adults because bone biopsies are rarely conducted unless specific blood tests indicate the condition.

Are You at Risk?

Medical science does not fully understand why some people lose bone mass more rapidly than others, but there are general risk factors:

- Being female
- Inadequate dietary calcium
- A family history of osteoporosis
- Early menopause
- Inactive lifestyle
- Petite build and low body weight
- Medications that include thyroid replacement, steroids
- Smoking and high alcohol consumption
- Celiac disease

What Causes Bone Loss in Celiac Disease?

It was once thought that the low bone density and osteoporosis so common in celiac disease were due to the malabsorption of calcium and vitamin D. It is now understood that the mechanism of bone loss in celiac disease is more complex. In addition to the risk factors listed above, many interacting factors can rob bone of its mass and density in celiac disease.

Malabsorption

Low bone density and osteoporosis in celiac disease can in fact be caused by calcium, vitamin D, or magnesium malabsorption. In particular, patients with severe diarrhea may have equally severe vitamin and mineral deficiencies.

If vitamin D is malabsorbed, it compounds the malabsorption of calcium. Vitamin D is derived from two main sources: the diet (as a fat-soluble vitamin) and the skin (through the action of sunlight). Malabsorption of vitamin D may be an issue, particularly in elderly, housebound patients who rarely venture into the sun. People are also spending less time sunbathing because of the cancer risks.

Magnesium also affects calcium absorption, and a deficiency can worsen its malabsorption. This can be corrected as the body uses only tiny amounts of magnesium. It is rarely given as a single supplement; larger doses than needed can cause diarrhea.

Failure to Obtain Maximum Bone Density in Childhood

It is now understood that patients who went undiagnosed for many years (or who believed they had "outgrown" celiac disease) often suffered from calcium malabsorption starting in childhood. This compromises bone formation and growth at its onset. The lack of necessary calcium may continue through adolescence and young adulthood when bone is forming its highest density, and into menopause, exacerbating the effects of normal aging when bone normally begins to thin. These patients are at particular risk to develop osteopenia and osteoporosis. They may already have it when the normal decline of bone mass starts in early adulthood.

Secondary Hyperparathyroidism

Bone remodeling is controlled by different hormones, the key one produced by the parathyroid gland. Normal blood levels of calcium are controlled by the *parathyroid hormone (PTH)*, which keeps blood calcium within a narrow, normal range. When calcium is needed—i.e., blood calcium levels are low—PTH is turned on. When levels are normal or high, it is turned off. This feedback mechanism is typically how hormones act.

Low calcium levels in the bloodstream due to malabsorption will turn on PTH—but at a price. Calcium is continually drawn out of the bones. This is a condition known as secondary hyperparathyroidism—PTH is continually and excessively secreted as an appropriate response to inadequate calcium absorption. This increases the breakdown of bone tissue and leads to bone loss. (See Parathyroid Hormone [PTH], page 115.)

Premature Menopause

Patients with celiac disease often enter menopause earlier than the general population. Hormone levels that stimulate bone regrowth drop, and this, in turn, can precipitate bone loss.

Genetic Predisposition

Bone size and structure have a genetic component—we resemble our parents, grandparents, or great-aunt Tillie. A family history of osteoporosis is a predisposing factor for the condition. If you are genetically prone to osteoporosis and have celiac disease in your family, you can skip immediately to Management Issues.

In men with celiac disease, low levels of male sex hormones (testosterone) will also result in further reduction in bone growth.

Inflammation

It is possible that the low bone density seen in patients with celiac disease may be related to the inflammatory process itself. Cytokines and other inflammatory mediators that arise from the inflamed small intestine circulate in the blood (see Chapter 2) and may affect bone formation by attacking bone tissue.

Autoimmunity

It has been demonstrated that patients with celiac disease have antibodies to "self" (autoantibodies). (See Chapter 14.) Autoantibodies are directed against a person's own tissue—they mistake our own body cells for foreign cells—and attack and destroy the perceived invader.

Tissue transglutaminase (tTG) (see What Is Tissue Transglutaminase [tTG]?, Chapter 2), the autoantibody that acts on gliadin in the gut, is also found in bone tissue and elsewhere, as in the skin. It is believed that a similar autoimmune reaction may contribute to the breakdown of bone in celiac disease. That is, antibodies to tTG will block the actions of tTG in bone, where it has important functions in remodeling.

The theory that ongoing gliadin ingestion may continually trigger these autoantibodies offers an interesting explanation for the bone deterioration in celiac disease. It may explain why low bone density and osteoporosis are common in the disease when many patients do not have malabsorption.

Management Issues

Managing low bone density, osteopenia, and osteoporosis in celiac disease is dependent on numerous factors, including age, family history, and severity of the situation in a given patient. Nonetheless, all adult patients diagnosed with celiac disease need to be tested to determine whether their bones will stand up.

Tests

BLOOD TESTS. All patients diagnosed with celiac disease should have blood work to assess their blood calcium, vitamin D, and PTH levels. These tests will indicate any potential for ongoing malabsorption of calcium or vitamin D.

URINARY CALCIUM. Patients who, when diagnosed, already have a low bone mineral density should also have their urinary calcium monitored with a twenty-four-hour urine excretion test. This test indicates how much calcium you are absorbing and how much of the calcium you are eating is being retained by your body.

BONE MINERAL DENSITY (BMD). A bone mineral density test is advised for all newly diagnosed adult celiac disease patients (male *and* female). A machine scans the hip, spine, and wrist bones and a patient's bones are compared with standardized norms set for their age, sex, and body size. If the bone density is considered below average, repeat scans are usually conducted every one to three years to monitor improvement on various dietary and supplement regimes.

Bone Mineral Density for Children

Measuring the bone mineral density of children with celiac disease is not as straightforward. The main problem is that standards to interpret the results are being determined only now. Adult standards are not applicable to children and adolescents who have not yet reached peak bone mass. A recent study outlined a new algorithm (method) being developed that, hopefully, will eliminate the diagnosis of osteoporosis often given when a child is evaluated using adult norms.

Bone Matrix Scanner

Bone density scans are routinely conducted with dual-energy X-ray absorptiometry (DXA). These machines are the current gold standard for assessing bone mineral density. They are used to predict the risk of fracture and to guide therapy for prevention of osteoporosis. Unfortunately, recent studies are showing that half of the fractures in post-menopausal women occur in those with bone density above the World Health Organization's diagnostic threshold for osteoporosis. It is becoming apparent that more detail is needed about the quality of our bones.

Therefore, a new generation of scanners has been developed that measures not only bone density but also bone structure and matrix. The test involves a CT of the wrist and ankle (a noninvasive procedure) and produces a precise three-dimensional snapshot of bone quality. The machine actually analyzes microstructure and connectivity—details that correlate with bone strength. In effect, doctors are able to visualize the supporting beams and crossbars of the building in addition to the condition of its bricks, mortar, and plaster. It is believed that this test will eventually be a better predictor of bone strength and fracture risk. Studies are now underway to validate its effectiveness.

The Effect of the Gluten-Free Diet

The first-line treatment for reduced bone density in celiac disease is a gluten-free diet and calcium supplements, with or without vitamin D. This enables the intestine to rebuild itself and normalize calcium, vitamin D, and magnesium absorption. Removing gluten from the diet also removes the toxic protein that initiates the autoimmune and inflammatory response in the body that appears to affect bone degeneration. Bone density will usually increase on this regimen.

The good news is that children with celiac disease are likely to fully regain a normal bone mass on a gluten-free diet. Unfortunately, this is often not the case with their adult counterparts. Adults with untreated celiac disease tend to have a lower bone mass and more problems rebuilding it, even when on a gluten-free diet.

We reach our maximum bone density in our twenties and rebuilding bone after that is difficult. Adults normally require a more active and intense program to rebuild what has been lost. While a gluten-free diet alone may not normalize bone mass in adults, it is still crucial to interrupt the destructive autoimmune inflammatory process.

Diet and Supplements

All patients with osteopenia and/or osteoporosis must be on a calcium-rich and balanced diet. A calcium-rich diet is the most effective way of supplying biologically available (more fully digestible) calcium to the body. Patients with celiac disease who have osteopenia or osteoporosis should discuss calcium supplements with their doctor. It is important to remember that calcium requires vitamin D to be effectively absorbed.

DAILY CALCIUM AND VITAMIN D RECOMMENDATIONS

Adults

Male–800–1,200 milligrams calcium/day;
400 IU vitamin D/day

Female–Premenopause (mid-twenties to early fifties)
1,000 milligrams calcium/day; 600 IU vitamin D/day

Female–Menopause (early fifties to late sixties)
1,000–1,200 milligrams calcium/day; 600 IU
vitamin D/day

Female–Postmenopause (late sixties, early seventies and
beyond)
1,000–1,200 milligrams calcium/day; 800 IU vitamin D/day

The body cannot properly absorb more than 500 to 600 milligrams of calcium at a time. While some excess is stored, most is eliminated. **This means that you should not take all your daily calcium supplements in one dose.** It is the equivalent of throwing them directly into the toilet.

Children with celiac disease should be treated with a gluten-free diet alone and supplemented only after consultation with their pediatrician.

Bone Resorption Agents

Adult patients with established osteoporosis may also require drugs that help to stimulate, build, and/or maintain bone mass. Antiresorption agents work to build and maintain bone mass by preventing the breaking-down process. Essentially, they block calcium from leaving bone and entering the bloodstream.

People with active celiac disease need to be aware that the antiresorptive drugs (e.g., Fosamax, Actonel) can cause serious side effects if given before the intestine is healed. As described earlier, calcium is so integral to muscle, nerve, and metabolic function that the body carefully maintains blood calcium at specific levels. If a patient has *active* celiac disease and inadequate calcium absorption from the gut, the body compensates and protects itself by limiting excretion and increasing bone breakdown. In essence, bones give to the body what the gut cannot. This maintains blood calcium at a normal level, but increases the loss of calcium from bone. Bone density falls, leading to osteoporosis.

When antiresorptive drugs are given that block the breakdown of bone, they can potentially block the main source of blood calcium for a celiac disease patient. Blood calcium can drop to dangerous levels. That, in turn, may cause cardiac arrythmias, muscle weakness, and convulsions. It is, therefore, important not to blockade the skeletal supply for blood calcium before the intestine is able to compensate and absorb calcium normally.

If the bone density has not improved sufficiently after at least a year on the diet and calcium supplements, an antiresorptive agent may be considered. Newly diagnosed patients with low bone mineral density and little or no intestinal malabsorption problems may be started on antiresorptive therapy sooner.

Parathyroid Hormone (PTH)

PTH turns on the metabolic pathway that activates bone resorption (breakdown) and the movement of calcium into the bloodstream. In an interesting biochemical reversal, when PTH is given intermittently in low doses, a totally different pathway is turned on. The building process is activated, and bone is formed. Biochemical work on the specific pathways has progressed to the point where PTH is used in some osteoporotic patients to rebuild bone.

This form of therapy carries risks similar to those of the antiresorptive agents in patients with active celiac disease and malabsorption. PTH agents (such as Forteo) are advised only once blood levels of PTH and vitamin D are normal, blood levels and urinary excretion of calcium are normal, and secondary hyperparathyroidism has been ruled out or corrected and the patient has been on a gluten-free diet for at least a year.

Exercise

No discussion of osteoporosis is complete without the "E" word. The adage "use it or lose it" is especially appropriate where bone is concerned: exercise builds bone.

The overwhelming evidence and statistics that connect celiac disease to osteopenia and osteoporosis make a compelling case for prevention as well as early screening for the conditions. Early diagnosis and therapy are critical to permit patients with celiac disease to achieve normal peak bone mass and then maintain it.

Osteoporosis is a degenerative and sometimes crippling disease that can be effectively managed and potentially prevented in patients with celiac disease.

> My osteoporosis has reversed. My hemoglobin is normal. If I take care of it, future issues won't be a problem. It's a shame that so many people live with it and go undiagnosed. (Lori, 31)

10

Depression

*I would wake up in the morning, open my eyes, look at the clock,
and go back to sleep. I didn't want to get out of bed and face...
anything. It felt like a weight or a blanket on my brain. All my joints
ached. First it was one day a week, then two, then...more bad
days than good ones. I was always snapping—Mrs. Irritability. And I
was always dead tired.*

*The doctor said my headaches were migraines and gave me
medicine, my joint pain was muscular and put me on Advil, and
concluded that my thyroid medicine was dosed properly so I really
shouldn't be so dead tired all the time.*

*A year into this he said: "Look, you're obviously stressed. Do
you want some Prozac?" Stressed?! I felt awful, was always tired,
barked louder than the dog at everyone and everything, and he's
telling me it's all in my head?!*

*Sad thing is, I began to believe it. I saw different specialists for
eight years before (someone) made the celiac disease connection.*
(Anonymous, 49)

Recently, in a crowded auditorium of celiac patients, the question was
raised: "Prior to diagnosis, how many of you were told your symptoms
were stress- or depression-related?" Over three-quarters of the attendees raised their hands.

*If I had a broken leg, you could see why I can't walk. But you can't
see inside my brain to see why I can't think. You can't see why I feel
the way I do.* (Sally, 23)

Every year, depression affects seventeen to eighteen million people in the United States.* For many, the symptoms of depression are severe enough to impact every aspect of their school, work, social, and/or home lives. Depression knows no age boundaries, although women are twice as likely as men to suffer its effects.

Depression is quite common among people with *any* chronic illness, and celiac disease is no exception. Unfortunately, it is difficult to determine if depression is a separate condition or a result of having celiac disease. The key issue is whether celiac disease actually causes depression. And is it possible to separate the two in the setting of a chronic inflammatory disease? The medical criteria for and definitions of depression only add to the diagnostic conundrum.

What Is Depression?

I went from Librium to Valium to Prozac. Nothing worked. One doctor had the nerve to tell me: "You're entering menopause and going through an awful divorce: you should be depressed." (Anonymous, 52)

Depression can be hard to classify. It may cause changes in the way we think, the way we feel about ourselves and others, our emotions, our behaviors, and our sense of physical well-being. Depression can arise as a manifestation of a disease (reactive), exist as an independent condition, or be a combination of the two.

The essential features that define the condition are described in *The Diagnostic and Statistical Manual of Mental Disorders* (5th edition; American Psychiatric Association, 2013). The *DSM-V* is the standard classification of mental disorders used by mental health professionals in the United States. For each disorder included in the *DSM-V*, there is a set of diagnostic criteria that indicate what symptoms must be present (and for how long) in order for an individual to qualify for a particular diagnosis. To be diagnosed with depression, a person must exhibit at least five symptoms that include:

- Persistent sad, anxious, or "empty" mood
- Feelings of hopelessness, pessimism
- Feelings of guilt, worthlessness

---

* www.nimh.nih.gov/depression

- A loss of interest in activities that were once enjoyed, including sex (*anhedonia*)
- Thoughts of death or suicide; suicide attempts
- Decreased energy, fatigue
- Difficulty concentrating, remembering
- Difficulty sleeping, changed sleep habits, or oversleeping
- Change in appetite—weight loss or gain
- Irritability, anger
- Persistent physical symptoms that do not respond to treatment—such as headaches, digestive disorders, and chronic pain

The last six symptoms in the above list dramatically illustrate the problem for patients with celiac disease: they describe a large percentage of patients with celiac disease prior to their diagnosis.

The *DSM-V* can provide criteria for a medical professional in the diagnosis of depression (or any other mental disorder). Unfortunately, it cannot determine the cause/effect relationship of any mental condition or rule out the potential for a patient to have both celiac disease and depression concurrently.

I kept thinking: I can handle this on my own. (Sandi, 44)

People with celiac disease regularly suffer through years of symptomatic illness before being diagnosed. The dilemma is that constant exhaustion, nagging joint pain, itchy dermatitis, stomachaches and bloating, headaches, and a long list of other symptoms can, in themselves, cause depression. There is no blood or pathology test for depression. Many patients become frustrated, depressed, angry, or lose hope of ever getting better because no one can "see" or measure their pain and therefore objectively determine if their illness is real.

My daughter would sit on my lap and cling to me while the other kids were playing. She always hung back. It was so unlike her. But she was otherwise healthy and happy. I decided to have her tested, since my youngest child had celiac disease. Her bloods were questionable, but the biopsy was totally flat! Her only symptom was this sudden inability to leave my side! (Sue, 41)

Children and adolescents also get depressed, but in this population it is often harder to separate illness and/or depression from normal mood swings and hormone changes. There are many processes that lead to depression, and the diagnosis and treatment of the condition in children and adolescents must be handled by a professional. Chronic illness in childhood requires appropriate treatment for both body and mind if the patient is to successfully handle both the illness and be able to navigate lifelong restrictions on diet and lifestyle. (For more on this subject, see Chapter 25.)

What Causes Depression in Celiac Disease?

One psychologist said to me: "Pain is very depressing to people."
My outlet is making fun of myself. Other days I sit down and cry.
(Anna, 40)

The precise mechanisms involved in the origins of mental and behavioral disorders in people with celiac disease are not known. A number of connections have been explored in various studies:

1. *Depression and celiac disease exist independently as separate conditions in the same patient.* This can occur prior to and/or after diagnosis. When two statistically common conditions occur in a general population, it is hard to determine if there is a causal relationship.

2. *Depression may be a reaction to the illness,* resulting from years of chronic, painful symptoms, of never feeling well.

   I tried to explain to my doctor that I was depressed because I never felt well, not the other way around. (Anonymous, 39)

   There are many psychological manifestations to any chronic disease that goes undiagnosed and untreated for years. Some studies showed that anxiety and depression are considered to be a reaction to chronic disease conditions and not a personality component. There are also studies in inflammatory bowel disease that indicate that the depression is reactive to the illness.

   Stress may also predispose to, precipitate, or maintain depression in people. Chronic stress is known to impact the immune system. It affects the body's ability to fight off infections, and it changes the mix of various white blood cells that circulate in the bloodstream and aid in healing. The old wives' tale that depressed and highly stressed people come down with more colds/flu has a physiological basis.

3. *Depression may be reactive to the restrictive lifestyle of celiac disease.* One study concluded that there is a possibility that some of the depression observed in patients with celiac disease could be related to the restrictive dietary and lifestyle aspects of the disease—and that patients who receive the diagnosis as adults are more likely to be challenged by the sudden need to change food and lifestyle habits. Teenagers and adults may also fear being identified as "sick" or "different" from others and lose their role, image, and place in society.

I think I had a harder time dealing with the diagnosis than I imagined.... It was a major lifestyle change—I told my mom: "I can't do this." And it became very difficult ... it affected things socially.

The food issues have become a more emotional point. Like trying to find a restaurant my friends and I can all go to. When they order Chinese, I don't order that night. I think my friends eat pizza less often now—which is better from a dietary point of view. It is difficult walking along the streets and smelling it. My friends try to be as accommodating as possible, but it's not their problem.

I think I withdrew more because it was very hard to be among my friends who were eating everything I wanted to be eating and couldn't be eating. I found myself eating alone more. (Melanie, 22)

This fear of rejection—by family, friends, waiters, work associates—led participants in one study to (a) irritability, and (b) a greater "conformism" and increased desire for social acceptance.

This study, and others, emphasized the need for a greater understanding of the psychological effects of the celiac disease diagnosis.

4. *Depression may be due to the malabsorption of nutrients.* One study suggested that malabsorption could interfere with the neurotransmitters that regulate mood. Researchers found a possible link between brain function, depression, and malabsorption because of abnormalities in the metabolism of *monoamines* (serotonin, dopamine, noradrenaline). They felt that a high number of food factors are involved in monoamine synthesis and concluded that the depression and anxiety disturbances found in celiac disease and IBD could be secondary to a reduced neural production of monoamines.

Nutrient Malabsorption—Folic Acid

A deficiency of folate (folic acid) was shown to increase irritability and forgetfulness. Folic acid is a vitamin that is necessary for the formation and growth of blood cells and is used in cell division. A deficiency plays a role in neurological defects in newborns, anemia, blood disorders, and GI disturbances, and was proved to cause depressive symptoms including fatigue and apathy.

Since folic acid is best absorbed in the duodenum, people with celiac disease may suffer from a deficiency. The link between this and depression is unclear, but interesting.

The malabsorption of other nutrients may contribute to depression. Vitamin B_{12} deficiency will also contribute to depression as well as dementia (memory problems). Once the intestine has healed, absorption improves, and the effects of these deficiencies should resolve.

5. *Depression may be related to thyroid or adrenal disorders.* Patients with hypothyroidism have relatively high rates of depression. Neuroendocrine abnormalities have been extensively studied as a way to open a "window to the brain" regarding the development of depression. It was reported that depressed patients have had alterations in thyroid stimulation/response mechanisms, and an abnormally high rate of antithyroid antibodies. (See Thyroid Disease, Chapter 14.)

   There is considerable controversy regarding what comes first in this scenario. That is, do alterations in endocrine secretion contribute directly to depression or do the altered secretions contribute to the signs and symptoms of an existing disorder. The large number of people with both celiac disease and thyroid disease makes this an interesting area of exploration.

6. *Depression is related to the inflammatory (i.e., immune) response in celiac disease.* Fatigue and depression are associated with the activation of the inflammatory response. In fact, the body's response to illness—the so-called sickness response—is to lock and barricade the doors. People take to their beds, shiver, run fevers, sleep a great deal—all in order to enable the body to fight off the bug or infection and heal. Prolonged illness produces a prolonged "sickness response" and depression may be related to the biological processes needed to heal.

One study suggested that the conservation-withdrawal reaction that occurs during prolonged threat to the body may access the same neural circuits that are involved in the processes that do cause depression (e.g., loss of a loved one, negative self-image).

The inflammatory agents implicated in several studies were the cytokines that are involved in the immune response of the body. These proteins are an integral part of the immune-inflammatory reaction. High levels of pro-inflammatory cytokines have been shown to:

- Induce abnormalities of thyroid hormone concentrations
- Induce behavioral alterations that resemble some symptoms of depression
- Affect many different organ functions such as bone formation

There appears to be some evidence that cytokine levels outside the brain may cause changes in cytokine expression and activity in the brain. Interestingly, some antidepressants impair the release of pro-inflammatory cytokines and enhance the expression of anti-inflammatory cytokines.

Research data supports the view that depression is characterized by both neuroendocrine and immune changes in the body. Current research is targeting immune sites in the search for new antidepressants that increase anti-inflammatory cytokine production (versus pro-inflammatory cytokines).

The relationship of the brain and the intestine is currently under intense study. The major class of antidepressants now in use is the *selective serotonin reuptake inhibitor (SSRI)*. The desired effect of these antidepressants is in the brain, but the bulk of the serotonin that is found in the body is, in fact, in the intestine! There are many fascinating areas for research in the area of biological psychiatry.

7. *Genetic influence.* Genes also play a role in depression. A family history of depression is a significant risk factor for depression in general and among children and adolescents with a chronic illness. Since genes also play a large role in celiac disease, it is possible that the two risks overlap in certain families.

The Effect of the Gluten-Free Diet

After two weeks on the diet, her whole personality changed—I said:
"Who are you?"
The mood change was dramatic; that was the first big change.
The second change was her ability to enjoy herself; she was able to
get up for classes. She still loves to sleep, but she's capable of get-
ting up now. (Mother of college student with celiac disease)

While the causes of depression in celiac disease may not be clear-cut, the effect of a gluten-free diet for some patients is quite striking. Many patients describe a constant, often overwhelming anxiety, memory loss, and grieflike depression that gets better on a gluten-free diet. Others talk of "the clouds disappearing" and the "fogginess" going away. While there is no science behind these observations, similar responses are often heard.

Interestingly, some patients find the restrictiveness of the diet itself to be a cause of ongoing depression. Reactions to the diet and the diagnosis may also include anxiety. Having a serious medical condition that requires lifelong dietary and lifestyle restrictions can provoke many different psychological responses. Some people choose to follow overly restrictive or hypervigilant diets, which can lead to high levels of anxiety and a lower quality of life. (See Hypervigilance, Chapter 26.)

While a preponderance of attendees at a recent support group spoke of having depression at some point during and/or after their diagnosis, many felt that the diet cleared up a great deal of their psychological symptoms.

The Bottom Line

None of the possible mechanisms behind depression in celiac disease are exclusive of one another. And it is almost impossible to separate "state" from "separate illness" in a manner that will apply to all patients. What is depressing for one is simply an annoyance for another.

The initial response of the doctor diagnosing celiac disease strongly influences the response of the patient. A strong patient-doctor relationship helps patients understand and accept the diagnosis. Physicians and other professionals should be aware of the psychological evaluation required for patients with celiac disease.

There are a number of interesting connections between belly and brain that are explored more fully in *Gluten Exposed*.

11

Dermatitis Herpetiformis and Other Skin Diseases

I now refer to it as my "seven-year itch." The itching was so bad I wanted to scratch my bones. It kept me awake at night. I wore long-sleeved shirts and pants in ninety-five-degree heat to cover the outbreaks. Numerous creams and lotions did not stop the itch that was increasingly consuming my waking hours. There was a certain irony as I used both left and right hands to scratch the mirrorlike eruptions in tandem.

The ultimate conclusion as to the cause of my "unexplained dermatitis" was "stress." Since our skin is a living, breathing organ that is affected by both our physical and mental health, that began to make sense to my grumpy, sleep-deprived brain. After seven years of itching, joint pain, and constant fatigue, if nothing else, I was definitely stressed. (Rory Jones)

Dermatitis herpetiformis (DH) is celiac disease of the skin. The eruptions, like the varied symptoms of celiac disease, are often mistaken for and treated as other skin conditions. Patients with dermatitis herpetiformis routinely see numerous dermatologists without getting the proper diagnosis. They are diagnosed—or dismissed—with mosquito bites, infected mosquito bites, eczema, contact dermatitis, allergies, heat and/or cold reaction, diabetic pruritus, psoriasis, hives, nerves, or "unexplained dermatitis," the ultimate catchall. Some patients get a label of recurrent herpes—as the name implies, the rash of dermatitis herpetiformis appears "herpetic." Topical creams and ointments mask symptoms and eruptions that can cover more and more of the body.

If celiac disease is the "masquerader" of digestive diseases—undiagnosed and often obscure to both patient and doctor—dermatitis herpetiformis is simply off most dermatological radar screens.

> *I am seventy-nine years old and I was just diagnosed with dermatitis herpetiformis. All my life I was undiagnosed by doctors and specialists who told me I had mosquito bites, flea bites, pruritus from diabetes, psoriasis, hives, etc., etc., etc. My dermatologist gave me ultraviolet light treatments for two years and that didn't help.*
>
> *My father, his mother, her father, and one of my brothers all had celiac disease; my father and brother had it as children and thought that they "grew out of it"—but I don't think so.*
>
> *I recently got awful diarrhea and, being a librarian, started to do research and asked my internist if I had celiac/sprue and started to treat myself with a gluten-free diet.* It took a bit, but I've finally stopped scratching! (Joan, 79)*

Of the two million or more patients currently diagnosed with celiac disease, approximately 10 percent are believed to have dermatitis herpetiformis. (Some studies show this figure to be higher.) In contrast with celiac disease, males with the condition outnumber females 2:1. The average age of onset for the disease is between twenty-five and forty-five years—dermatitis herpetiformis rarely affects adolescent or prepubescent children. This delayed onset indicates that long-term stimulation of the immune system by gluten is needed to produce the symptoms of dermatitis herpetiformis.

Studies also showed that approximately 20 to 30 percent of patients with dermatitis herpetiformis have thyroid abnormalities, and many do not have any gastrointestinal symptoms. In fact, the skin manifestation does not correlate with intestinal severity or damage. Some people (about 20 percent) with dermatitis herpetiformis actually have normal small intestine biopsies.

---

* We do not recommend starting a gluten-free diet based on self-diagnosis.

What Is Dermatitis Herpetiformis?

I'm itching to death. (Becky)

Dermatitis herpetiformis was first described by Dr. Louis Duhring in 1884, four years before Samuel Gee made sense of the "coeliac affliction." In 1967 Janet Marks of England discovered the link between intestinal biopsy results and skin biopsy results of dermatitis herpetiformis patients.

Dermatitis herpetiformis is characterized by an intensely itchy, blistering rash. The textbooks say that it occurs on extensor surfaces (e.g., elbows and knees). But clinically it can occur anywhere, including limbs, trunk, groin, hands, fingers, face, scalp, and along the hairline. Most patients scratch the itchy skin until it breaks or bleeds; therefore, the outbreak often looks like a rash with *excoriations* (abraded skin caused by scratching).

> *They told me I had jock itch. It's not like you can scratch yourself there around other people, and sometimes the itch was so awful I didn't know what to do with myself.* (Anonymous, 35)

The blisters tend to recur in the same place each time and are mirrored on both sides of the body. The itching and burning insinuates itself into every aspect of a person's life—interrupting sleep, work, and play. Some patients report that sweating during an exercise session can irritate the blisters. Unfortunately, scratching further irritates the blisters and can cause scarring.

People do not "itch to death," so it is often hard for people with dermatitis herpetiformis to explain adequately their suffering to family, friends, and doctors. The physical blisters, continual scratching, and concurrent loss of sleep take a psychological toll on many patients. In the nineteenth century, before systemic drugs were introduced that alleviated the itching, dermatitis herpetiformis was reported as a cause of suicides.

Dermatitis herpetiformis is a chronic, permanent condition if not treated with a gluten-free diet. Patients may or may not ever develop gastrointestinal symptoms. Some patients suffer from many of the same malabsorption problems as people who have celiac disease without dermatitis herpetiformis (e.g., osteoporosis, anemia), and they may require treatment from specialists other than the diagnosing dermatologist.

How Do I Know If I Have It—
Tests for Dermatitis Herpetiformis

The diagnosis of dermatitis herpetiformis is made based on:

- The historical occurrence and appearance of a blistering rash and/or scabbed lesions
- Confirmation by a skin biopsy

Blood tests for celiac disease—notably endomysial antibodies (EMA) and antitissue transglutaminase (tTG) may be positive or even negative in patients with dermatitis herpetiformis. Up to 30 percent of those with dermatitis herpetiformis will not have these antibodies, since they correlate with the severity of the small intestinal lesion and not the severity of the skin lesion. Patients with a minimal, or no detectable, lesion in the intestine will have negative blood tests for celiac disease.

There is a definite spectrum of sensitivity to gluten in those with dermatitis herpetiformis, and some people are exquisitely sensitive to even trace amounts. The occurrence of lesions after an ingestion of gluten (anywhere from several hours to several days) is another indication of the condition.

The gold standard for diagnosis (see Skin Biopsy, Chapter 4) is a skin biopsy of *uninvolved* skin adjacent to an eruption—best taken within millimeters of a lesion. The biopsy must be done by a knowledgeable dermatologist because a sampling of tissue from the eruption itself can be confused with other skin conditions. A biopsy of the actual lesion will give a characteristic appearance, but it is not possible to do the immunological staining that is necessary to make the diagnosis. This is because the inflammatory reaction in the blistering lesion destroys the early signs of the immune deposits that are still present in adjacent tissue.

The biopsy is tested for granular IgA (immunoglobulin A) deposits in the *dermal papillae* (under the top layer of skin) using direct immunofluorescence. The term *granular* refers to the pattern of immunofluorescence, a very specific appearance that differentiates dermatitis herpetiformis from another, almost identical disease, linear IgA disease. Patients do not need a small bowel biopsy unless they have clinical manifestations of small bowel disease. **If you have a positive diagnosis of dermatitis herpetiformis, you have celiac disease. And you must**

adhere to a gluten-free diet no matter how "normal" your intestine may appear.

Since no tests in medicine are 100 percent, not everyone with dermatitis herpetiformis will have a positive skin biopsy. A negative biopsy should not necessarily be used to exclude the diagnosis if the lesions look and act like dermatitis herpetiformis and occur after the ingestion of gluten. Patients should be retested, making sure that both the lab technique and specimen taken are appropriate for determining the diagnosis.

Dermatitis herpetiformis biopsies for IgA are usually positive for a long time after gluten has been stopped—and become positive again within a few months of ingesting gluten. But, it is unclear what dose of gluten is necessary.

Because of the intense itching and discomfort, many patients with dermatitis herpetiformis are unwilling to undergo a gluten challenge to be retested. (For details, see Gluten Challenge, Chapter 4.) But since even small amounts of gluten may trigger an almost immediate response on the skin, this may be attempted.

Dermatitis herpetiformis should not be self-diagnosed. If pathology is negative, the diagnosis should be reviewed by a dermatologist or physician knowledgeable about the condition.

Where Does It Come From—Pathogenesis

Dermatitis herpetiformis, like celiac disease, has a multifactorial derivation. It requires:

- A genetic predisposition
- Prolonged exposure to gluten—the protein in wheat, rye, and barley
- An immunological response

In susceptible individuals, the chronic stimulation of the immune system by gluten produces IgA antibodies that bind to the skin and cause dermatitis herpetiformis. Tissue transglutaminase (tTG) (see What Is Tissue Transglutaminase [tTG]?, Chapter 2)—the enzyme that is integrally involved in setting off the reactions that destroy the villi in celiac disease—may also play a role. There are many different forms of tissue transglutaminase found in the body. The form of the enzyme found in the skin (epidermal transglutaminase) appears to cross-react with IgA antibodies and set off the chain reaction that causes the inflammation, itching, and blistering of dermatitis herpetiformis. As researchers learn more about the immune reactions of epidermal transglutaminase, therapies may be developed to block the response.

Dermatitis Herpetiformis and Other Diseases

Patients with dermatitis herpetiformis have a higher incidence of non-Hodgkin's lymphoma than the general population. The gluten-free diet reduces the risk. Patients with dermatitis herpetiformis also have a higher incidence of anemia and other autoimmune diseases such as thyroid disease, type 1 diabetes, lupus, Sjögren's syndrome, and vitiligo (see page 134). This is a similar scenario to that of patients with celiac disease in the absence of dermatitis herpetiformis—not surprising, since they are the same condition.

Skin diseases seem to occur commonly in people with dermatitis herpetiformis and celiac disease. Patients can also develop more than one condition, which can be confusing. In particular, there are forms of eczema that look (and itch) just like dermatitis herpetiformis lesions, and the blisters can be confused without biopsy confirmation.

Bruising

There is also a bruising phenomenon that occurs with celiac disease. This can be due to three different factors:

- Malabsorption of vitamin K, resulting in coagulation problems, bleeding, and bruising
- *Idiopathic thrombocytopenic purpura (ITP)*, an autoimmune reaction against the platelets resulting in bruising and bleeding
- Scurvy, due to a lack of vitamin C and resulting in fragile capillaries and bruising

Management Issues

The current treatment of dermatitis herpetiformis is based on the following:

1. A strict adherence to a gluten-free diet
2. The use of medications to relieve the itching and burning of the blisters

Systemic Drugs

The main drug used to treat dermatitis herpetiformis is dapsone (sulfa-pyridine is also effective). In use for many years, dapsone blocks the inflammatory process in the skin lesions, but it does not affect the IgA deposits under the dermis or the ongoing immune response. For unknown reasons, the facial lesions of some patients may not respond as well to the drug.

Unfortunately, some patients use dapsone's effectiveness in controlling their symptoms as a license to cheat on the diet. Nevertheless, dapsone only *suppresses* itching and the lesions themselves; it should not be used to replace a gluten-free diet or as an excuse for noncompliance. It is a drug with some potentially serious side effects that must be monitored by a physician and used in the lowest possible doses, for the shortest possible period of time. Side effects include hemolytic anemia, leukopenia, headaches, peripheral neuropathy, kidney damage, and fatigue. Any patients going on dapsone therapy must have their blood levels checked for G6PD deficiency prior to starting the drug and must be monitored for the development of anemia.

It is very important that patients do not receive systemic steroids for the rash. Although steroids will alleviate the itch, high doses of steroids are necessary for such an outcome. Patients with dermatitis herpetiformis, as with celiac disease, have a high rate of bone problems, and the use of steroids can aggravate bone loss.

Topical Creams

Topical creams containing cortisone (steroids) are also prescribed to alleviate symptoms. Used for prolonged periods of time, these creams also cause complications. They can thin the skin and, when overused, cause ancillary rashes due to the breaking of superficial blood vessels.

Other creams such as tacrolimus (Protopic) and pimecrolimus (Elidel) also alleviate symptoms. These drugs are referred to as "immune modulators" and work by suppressing the immune system. When used topically, they do not weaken or change the body's immune system, do not have the side effects of topical steroids, and are indicated for eczema and other skin conditions as well.

None of the systemic or topical drugs eliminate the cause of the eruptions; they simply suppress or ease the symptoms—symptoms that will repeatedly recur until gluten is eliminated from the body.

*I'm on a gluten-free diet, and I'm still breaking out! When will the
itching stop?* (Jon, 39)

What Triggers Dermatitis Herpetiformis?

Dermatitis herpetiformis can be a very erratic disease. Since the skin
may not be rid of the IgA deposits for more than two years after starting
a gluten-free diet, it is possible to get flare-ups that arrive without obvious gluten ingestion. It is not uncommon for patients to experience
outbreaks of facial and scalp lesions while on dapsone *and* a gluten-free
diet. In fact, it may take patients a substantial amount of time to erase
years of IgA buildup in the skin. A flare-up could also be due to inadvertent gluten ingestion—even on a strict diet, it can "slip" in. But, there
are other ingested substances that may also play a role in flare-ups.

Iodine

*There was a raw bar at the party, and I was going for the world io-
dine record. Raw also described my face and hands the next day.*
(Jon, 39)

There appears to be an intimate relation between dermatitis herpetiformis
and iodine. It is unclear what the mechanism of this relationship is, but we
do know that people who have dermatitis herpetiformis also appear to be
sensitive to iodine. Often the dermatitis herpetiformis will not improve—
and flare-ups may occur—unless iodine is minimized or eliminated from
the diet. This includes iodized salt or salty foods (pretzels, chips, etc.—
gluten-free, of course), and different forms of seafood. Sushi may be a real
issue due to the high amount of iodine in seaweed. After the dermatitis herpetiformis lesions have resolved, iodine may be reintroduced to the diet.

NSAIDs

Nonsteroidal anti-inflammatory drugs (aspirin, ibuprofen) also seem to
aggravate lesions. Patients with dermatitis herpetiformis may want to
substitute acetaminophen for pain and aches if NSAIDs cause problems.

Skin Lotions/Creams/Hair Products

Another area of controversy—one of the "myths" that refuse to
disappear—is whether or not gluten can be absorbed through the skin.
Dermatologists who are experts on the topic say no, the only causes for

concern are the things that we ingest—and that includes lipstick, a cosmetic that is consumed by the pound.

Some support groups recommend eliminating any skin lotions or hair products that contain gluten sources. Unless you are eating these products (a hazard in its own right) they are not going to cause dermatitis herpetiformis. If skin lotions do cause rashes, you should consult a dermatologist or allergist to see what element of the lotion might be triggering the reaction. It is also possible that these products contain ingredients that irritate broken skin, a common side effect of healing dermatitis herpetiformis lesions.

Stress

Skin is the largest organ of the body and is linked directly to the brain. People become red-faced when angry and blush when embarrassed. Stress may be a factor in skin flare-ups of different types of dermatitis that are hard to distinguish from dermatitis herpetiformis. There is no science behind a dermatitis herpetiformis/stress link, but patients have reported an increase in symptoms under stressful conditions.

The Effect of the Gluten-Free Diet

The backbone of therapy for dermatitis herpetiformis is the gluten-free diet. It is the only "cure" for the condition. Unfortunately, when dermatitis herpetiformis does recur—through accidental or deliberate gluten ingestion—it has a life of its own. That is, one "insult" may take one to two weeks to clear up, whether or not there is any further gluten ingestion.

Patients with dermatitis herpetiformis need to be patient—and good patients—since the effects of a gluten-free diet may not be immediate. If you have had a skin disease for many years, it may take many years to get better.

Hiding in Plain Sight

Dermatitis herpetiformis is an almost unique example of the existence of "silent" celiac disease—if the profound itching that characterizes the condition can be considered silent. Most patients manifest and are diagnosed with dermatitis herpetiformis in their late twenties, thirties, and forties, which indicates an active disease process working for decades beneath the skin. The only way to extinguish the "itch that you cannot scratch" is to diagnose its source and remove gluten from the diet.

Other Skin Conditions

Eczema and Psoriasis

Both eczema and psoriasis, two fairly common skin conditions, are often found in patients with celiac disease and dermatitis herpetiformis.

Psoriasis is classified as an inflammatory autoimmune disease, although specific autoantibodies have not been identified. It is often seen in patients with celiac disease. The inflamed, red, and often patchy skin of psoriasis and eczema may mimic the symptoms of dermatitis herpetiformis. Although it is still being studied, a gluten-free diet does not influence the course of psoriasis. One study showed that a small percentage of patients with psoriasis had antigliadin antibodies (in the absence of celiac disease). In this study, those patients seemed to benefit from a gluten-free diet.

The gluten-free diet does not usually appear to have any impact on eczema, though some patients report improvement when following it.

Eczema and psoriasis can occur independently or concurrently with dermatitis herpetiformis. As noted before, patients with celiac disease and dermatitis herpetiformis seem to be prone to various forms of dermatitis—they often seem to "itch." Whether this is due to some underlying immunological response or simply the normal complement of allergies, dry skin, and stress-related rashes and bumps is unknown.

Vitiligo

Vitiligo is a skin disorder in which the *melanocytes* (the cells that make pigment in the skin) are destroyed. White, patchy areas of skin appear on parts of the body, and hair growing in those areas may appear white.

Vitiligo is an autoimmune condition associated with celiac disease. It is very common and affects all races, skin types, and ethnicities. About 1 to 2 percent of the worldwide population suffers from this disease, and most sufferers will develop it before their fortieth birthday.

Treatment traditionally consists of topical steroids and creams. In the past few years, effective new therapies involving narrow-band *ultraviolet B (UVB)* therapy has helped patients with moderate to severe vitiligo. Patients must wear sunscreen because the skin affected can be very easily burned when exposed to the sun.

The effect of the gluten-free diet is unclear.

The skin is a living, breathing organ that reflects the health of its owner. Nevertheless, it is sometimes difficult for both patient and doctor to make the necessary connections to the GI tract when a rash, bump, lesion, or itch appears. Dermatitis herpetiformis is a part of the celiac iceberg that is almost entirely under the waterline.

12

Diabetes

Man may be the captain of his fate, but he is also the victim of his blood sugar.

—Wilfred Oakley

I was diagnosed with diabetes in 1992, when I was nine and a half. I was not a big water drinker and I was drinking a ton. My mom was suspicious and took a urine sample to the pediatrician one morning while I was in school. The doctor said: "Where is she? Get her, she's going to the hospital." I was in the hospital for six days, learning about everything.

I had stomachaches more frequently than normal and thought: "If I can deal with the diabetes, I can deal with a stomachache." Things became much worse in high school. Senior year I was diagnosed with mono and anemia within a week of each other. I was out of school for weeks and lost ten to fifteen pounds. I was always tired. With the diabetes, it's like . . . what's a symptom, what's a problem?

In college I was sleeping eighteen hours a day and not going to classes because I was so tired. My mom . . . was very active in JDRF (Juvenile Diabetes Research Foundation) . . . and was learning more and more about celiac disease, and said why not get tested?

I had blood work and an endoscopy. Coming out of anesthesia, the doctor confirmed it: I had completely flattened villi. I was in a drugged state, but in shock. I think I had a harder time dealing with the celiac diagnosis than when I handled the diabetes. (Mel, 22)

There are approximately twenty-one million diagnosed and another eight million undiagnosed diabetics in the United States today.* Diabetes is the leading cause of new cases of blindness in people twenty to seventy-four and of end-stage renal (kidney) disease. It is also the most common cause of vascular disease.[†] About 1.25 million of the diagnosed diabetics are type 1, or insulin-dependent. And a recent study showed that 8 to 10 percent of this group will also develop celiac disease, usually within ten years of their diagnosis of diabetes. This is a significant statistic for both diabetics and the celiac disease community. People with celiac disease have the same risk for type 2 (non-insulin-dependent) diabetes as the rest of the general population—another sobering statistic, since almost eighteen million people in the United States are prediabetic.

The association between type 1 or insulin-dependent diabetes mellitus (IDDM) and celiac disease has been recognized for more than forty years. Many diabetes clinics and specialists screen for celiac disease in their diabetic patients. Others do not. They believe what one professional told the mother of a diabetic daughter suffering from multiple, unexplained symptoms (later diagnosed as celiac disease): "You people are always looking for problems."

However, the restrictions placed on patients—especially children—with this double diagnosis are, in a word, challenging. They also put a large burden on the parents and family members of a child with IDDM and celiac disease.

When you're already feeling different, with so much beyond your control, the celiac disease is that much more difficult. (Mel, 22)

The initial learning curve may be steep, but navigating the "mountain of carbohydrates" and the double diet is well worth the effort. (For more on eating properly with diabetes or celiac disease, see Chapter 24.)

---

* American Diabetes Association
† American Diabetes Association

What Is Diabetes?

Diabetes (from the Greek *siphōn*, or "running through") mellitus ("sweet") is a lack or deficiency of insulin, the hormone that enables the body to use and store glucose (sugar). The definition literally describes a characteristic symptom of patients with the disease—the excretion of a large volume of glucose-filled urine.

Glucose is one dietary fuel that is critical for muscle and body function. In particular, the brain—which is active whether we are awake or asleep—relies almost exclusively on glucose for its continual energy needs. But, without insulin, the body is unable to use its most available source of energy—the glucose in food. Even as glucose builds to high levels in the bloodstream (*hyperglycemia*) after a meal, it cannot enter the cells that are famished for nourishment.

The kidneys, which normally reabsorb any glucose left in the bloodstream once insulin has finished its job, are unable to handle the increased glucose load and sugar spills into the urine (*glycosuria*). This, in turn, causes excess urine production, frequent urination, and increased thirst—all recognized signs of insulin deficiency/diabetes. The excess urine results in the loss of sodium and water, which can lead to dehydration causing low blood pressure (due to loss of blood volume) and brain dysfunction.

Literally "starving," the body begins to draw on fat and protein from the muscles for energy. This results in muscle wasting and weight loss. This emergency process releases excess fatty acids (in the form of *ketones*) into the bloodstream. They can cause the blood to become acidic and build up to a dangerous point (*ketoacidosis*), which can lead to coma or death.

There are two basic types of diabetes.

Type 1, or insulin-dependent diabetes mellitus (IDDM), formerly referred to as "juvenile onset" diabetes, is an autoimmune disorder that occurs mainly in younger people, but it can occur in adults. The immune system attacks and destroys the insulin-producing cells of the pancreas, setting off the sequence of events described above. When insulin is no longer produced by the body, it must be permanently replaced by insulin administered by injections or a pump.

Type 2, non-insulin-dependent diabetes mellitus (NIDDM), so-called "adult onset" diabetes, appears to start as an insulin resistance. That is, the insulin produced is less effective in controlling blood glucose. Type 2 diabetes is not an autoimmune condition, and insulin production is unstable, not absent. The condition appears to have a genetic or family association and occurs more commonly in older individuals who are also obese. However, it is increasingly being seen in overweight children whose cells cannot handle the amount of carbohydrates they are consuming.

Type 2 diabetics can often control their condition through diet alone or with oral (non-insulin) medications. Some will also require insulin shots for the control of blood glucose levels.

A third type—gestational diabetes—occurs during pregnancy and is usually temporary. The mother's body does not respond to insulin, and the condition can normally be controlled with diet alone. The condition usually resolves itself once the baby is born.

What Causes Type 1 Diabetes (IDDM)?

The ultimate destruction of islet cells (of the pancreas) in IDDM appears to be caused by numerous factors. The precise trigger is not as clear as the gliadin connection in celiac disease, but it may include:

- Autoimmune factors, antibodies that target the islet (beta) cells of the pancreas that produce insulin
- Infections (viruses) that attack the islet cells
- A miscommunication of antigen-presenting cells (APC) that cause killer T cells to target the islet cells—either the result of infections or autoimmune factors
- The development of celiac disease prior to IDDM

Diabetes and Celiac Disease

I was diagnosed with celiac disease Memorial Day weekend and went on a gluten-free diet. I was on the diet for two weeks and I lost four pounds. I attributed it to the Atkins effect.

Then, one day I was driving and couldn't read the license on the car in front of me. My vision had always been 20/40. The next week, I couldn't see my son on the soccer field. I was always starving, lost my vision, and was losing weight.

I now have IDDM (type 1 diabetes). I'm up to my head in new things. (Sara, 43)

In patients developing both celiac disease and diabetes, the diabetes is typically diagnosed first. The celiac disease may be discovered later because of a continuing failure to thrive in young children, lactose intolerance, bloating, diarrhea, unexplained weight loss, extreme fatigue, anemia, poor diabetic control, recurrent episodes of hypoglycemia, or because of screening.

Gastrointestinal symptoms are common in both diabetics and people with celiac disease: the overlap should not be ignored or written off as symptomatic of whichever condition was diagnosed first. Studies also showed that mild symptoms that are disregarded are often the ones recognized retrospectively.

A common scenario features the patient who is doing well on an insulin pump—maintaining his or her diet—whose blood sugar starts to ping-pong. This individual has more insulin than sugar in the bloodstream because the food he or she eats is not being absorbed. (See Chapter 2.) Low blood sugar brings the patient back to the doctor, who may adjust the insulin, assuming the patient does not need as much. He or she then eats a meal that is essentially gluten-free; more is absorbed and the glucose levels start running high. The ping-pong of glucose levels will often prompt a physician to test for celiac disease. Other patients, like Mel, report overwhelming fatigue.

There are currently no specific guidelines for diabetologists to follow regarding testing for celiac disease. Patients may not discuss symptoms such as bloating, which they consider to be normal and have had for as long as they can remember.

Nevertheless, the connection between celiac disease and diabetes has three well-defined links:

Genetic Predisposition

Both celiac disease and diabetes are associated with HLA-DQ2 and HLA-DQ8 genetic haplotypes. (See A Genetic Primer—Fitting the Groove, Chapter 6.) Further research is needed to pinpoint all of the specific genes responsible in these two conditions. And while these genes predispose, they do not determine the onset of either disease, separately or together.

The Mechanisms of Autoimmunity (T-Cell–Mediated Immune Reactions)

Children diagnosed with celiac disease were shown to have insulin autoantibodies and/or islet cell autoantibodies. These are antibodies implicated in the destruction of the pancreatic cells responsible for producing insulin (beta cells) and are also found in diabetics.

A recent study showed that celiac patients are at "high risk" of developing IDDM. Children with recently diagnosed celiac disease had a significantly higher prevalence of anti–islet cell and anti-insulin antibodies than nonceliacs. Researchers believe that during this period anti–islet cell antibodies serve as markers for future disease. The study demonstrated that children diagnosed with celiac disease who had anti–islet cell antibodies will lose them after starting a gluten-free diet. This suggests that the diagnosis and treatment of celiac disease prevented the development of diabetes.

Having One Autoimmune Disease Increases the Risk of Getting Another

Patients with celiac disease are at increased risk, beyond that of the general population, of developing other autoimmune disorders. The reasons are unclear, but autoimmune diseases seem to travel in groups. Conversely, patients with diabetes are also at higher risk to develop another autoimmune disease.

Some physicians have advocated the screening of all diabetics for celiac disease. There is evidence that treating celiac disease will prevent diabetes, but for those already diagnosed with type 1 diabetes, the horse is already out of the barn.

Management Issues

The dual management of diabetes and celiac disease involves the following:

- The control of blood sugar (glycemic control)
- The gluten-free diet and its relation to carb counting
- Recognizing and treating the complications of each disease
- Lifestyle and compliance issues

Glycemic Control

The medical aspects of diabetes and the specific needs of a diabetic patient are well covered through the American Diabetes Association, websites and books devoted to this topic, and the counseling of nutritionists and physicians.

Complications

Gastrointestinal symptoms and disturbances are also common in diabetics. This may be due to many different processes. *Gastroparesis*, the delayed emptying of the stomach (see When Normal Goes Pathological, Chapter 1), is seen in diabetics. It may be a manifestation of neuropathy (*diabetic autonomic neuropathy*) and can cause reflux, impaired digestion, recurrent vomiting, or a feeling of fullness. Most of the symptoms simply send people to the indigestion aisle in the drugstore. The gluten-free diet may resolve those symptoms if celiac disease is present and is the cause.

Diarrhea and constipation are common in diabetic patients—as well as general population. Diarrhea may be related to bacterial overgrowth due to stasis of the bowel or the result of disturbed motility. (See Chapter 3.) Diabetic neuropathy may affect the enteric nervous system (of the bowel), causing constipation. But celiac disease should also be considered if a patient has continuing GI symptoms.

Peripheral neuropathies are a common complication of diabetes as well as a common symptom of celiac disease. Dietary control and disease management are important to resolve both.

Lifestyle and Compliance Issues

I'm on an insulin pump that provides the best control of blood glucose levels. Using the pump, you continuously receive a basal level of insulin determined between you and your doctor. This basal level of insulin keeps your blood sugar at a normal level when you're not eating. Before each meal you program the pump to provide a bolus that covers what you'll be eating at that meal.

After using the pump for a while I know myself and how my body reacts to insulin; I know precisely that if I take one unit of insulin it will bring my blood glucose down 30 points. It's like clockwork. So you learn this about yourself as you live with the pump. When I eat rice pasta I know that since it contains a lot of carbohydrates it

*will bring my blood sugar up and so I take a little more insulin than I
would if I were just eating fish and vegetables.* (David, 51)

Patients with both celiac disease and type 1 diabetes not only must
avoid gluten, but must balance what and when they eat with their insulin needs and their level of activity. The glycemic response to many
gluten-free foods tends to be higher and faster. This may affect both insulin levels and an established dietary pattern. Many gluten-free foods
are higher in starch and sugar and lower in fiber than their wheat-based
counterparts (i.e., breads, waffles, cakes, cereals).

*There would be days when I'd go from nine A.M. to five P.M. and, if I
didn't have anything with me or (didn't) find something (gluten-free) for
lunch, I'd be waiting all day to eat. Since I wasn't eating, I wasn't testing my blood sugar as regularly because I usually test it before I eat. So
my control worsened, but sort of in an explainable way.* (Mel, 22)

While the dual diagnosis of celiac disease and type 1 diabetes affects all ages, it is typically newly diagnosed children, adolescents, and
young adults who have the greatest medical, dietary, and psychological
hurdles to overcome.

Adolescents and young adults in their twenties may have some of the
most difficult compliance issues, even without diabetes. Diabetes and
celiac disease require a certain amount of predictability—what, when,
and where you will be able to eat. The only predictable parts of most
teenage and twenty-something lives are last-minute plans, parties, work
deadlines, snacks, and activities. Each of them must learn to appreciate
the importance of compliance to both diets—and the price to be paid in
complications if they don't do so. **Any adolescent or young adult with a
chronic illness must buy into their own care.** For some patients, and
their families, this is an issue that may require professional assistance.
Many support groups also have teen meetings that offer peer assistance.

Adults may have an equally difficult time balancing the dual diets
and lifestyles.

Will I Get Better on a Gluten-Free Diet?

On a gluten-free diet, the intestine will begin to heal. For celiac disease
patients with severe GI symptoms, carbohydrates are now being absorbed
and can be monitored and metabolized by the insulin. While absorption

may vary until the gut is fully healed—requiring the adjustment of both the insulin taken and the carbs eaten—blood sugars should normalize and be easier to control within a few months.

Some studies showed that diabetic control improves on a gluten-free diet and that there are fewer hypoglycemic episodes. Others question this finding because of compliance issues.

The malabsorption of glucose may increase the risk of severe hypoglycemia in diabetics and frequent or severe hypoglycemia can affect neurologic function in diabetic children. Recurrent episodes of hypoglycemia should be a trigger to test for celiac disease.

The gluten-free diet will not cure someone already diagnosed with type 1 diabetes or reverse any of its complications. But studies indicate that autoantibodies do disappear on a gluten-free diet, and this may have a positive effect on someone with dual autoimmune diseases, especially children. A gluten-free diet is also necessary to guard against the long-term effects of celiac disease on the body. Growth patterns were shown to improve in diabetic children diagnosed with celiac disease. (See To Test or Not to Test, below.)

To Test or Not to Test

There is a great deal of controversy regarding the screening of non-symptomatic diabetic patients for celiac disease. Arguments for the testing include:

- The high prevalence of celiac disease in type 1 diabetics
- Early treatment (a gluten-free diet) can avert or reverse long-term complications such as osteoporosis/osteopenia, growth failure, and anemia
- Better glucose control

Arguments against testing include:

- The double diet requirements in asymptomatic patients can be burdensome and expensive.
- The dual diagnosis and diet carries a significant psychological burden.
- The long-term effects of asymptomatic or subclinical celiac disease are not well studied or known.

• Diabetics, as a group, do not have an increased risk of developing non-Hodgkin's lymphoma; therefore, this cannot be used as a reason to screen for, identify, or treat celiac disease.

Most clinicians advocate the testing of symptomatic patients—which includes all of the protean manifestations of celiac disease explained in Chapter 3.

> Diabetes was hard for me. When I was diagnosed, there were no glucose meters available. Just a test tape you had to pee on. There were a lot of problems with passing out in the middle of the night before glucose monitors for blood testing. That was pretty traumatic.
>
> There are diabetics who say: "One chocolate bar isn't going to kill me." They're fooling themselves. Once in a while is just as bad. A good number of well-educated people don't take charge and are letting themselves go. They're fainting and going into hypoglycemia.
>
> I really think that every child in the United States should be tested (for celiac disease). That's got to be a must. If it turns out that there's this diabetes link, that's what I'm really curious about, but who knows what other autoimmune disorders may be linked as well. If it's really true, then so much could be prevented by simply not eating gluten; it's worth a billion dollars.
>
> My advice? You can deal with it and live a perfectly normal life. I feel that I have no restrictions. Whether it be sports or traveling or going out to dinner or going to a wedding or whatever. There's just ways you can deal with it, and it's not traumatic or the end of the world.
>
> I'm not going to let it stop me. (David, 51)

Diabetes is one of the most common and most complicated associations with celiac disease. It requires a lifelong adherence to two restrictive diets and lifestyles. As with malignancies, the diabetes diagnosis usually outweighs the diagnosis of celiac disease, since there is a very high price to pay for noncompliance in the diabetic arena. Despite the restrictions, most patients can soon learn to enjoy a "living with," rather than "living without," lifestyle.

13

Infertility

I hated going to doctors—they always found something and it always turned out to be nothing. Occasionally I had elevated liver enzymes or anemia. Since college I had unexplained joint pain and fatigue—I had to sleep nine hours or I was toast.

I was over thirty-five and wanted to have a baby. After six months of trying I got tested and they told me: "Without intrauterine insemination or in vitro fertilization (IVF) you'll never get pregnant." I did two rounds of intrauterine insemination, then we went to IVF. It's quite an ordeal. You sit in this waiting room with dozens of other stressed-out females who are getting hormones and want to get pregnant.

My first pregnancy miscarried. Afterward, I got anemic and was exhausted. I was taking three-hour naps every day. I couldn't even walk around the block. I also had joint pain, and my internist said I had Lyme disease. I said: "I've had joint pain since 1985 and fatigue. It's not Lyme."

So I went to another local doctor who also tested me for Lyme and said it was negative, and he tacked on a test for celiac disease, which was positive. I said: "How do you spell celiac and gluten?" He recommended an endoscopy, which turned out positive.

I was going to do another IVF, and Dr. Green said: "Try the diet first for a while." I looked on a website, and it said that it took about two years for the gut to heal on a gluten-free diet and nothing will change (for pregnancy) for about nine months. I went on the diet and about that time I got night sweats, then they found out I had Graves' disease (hyperthyroidism). I had an allergic reaction to the *pills and got hives. It turned out one of the hives was squamous cell cancer.... I was looking down the wolf....*

Well, about nine months after I went on a gluten-free diet, practically to the day, I wasn't feeling well—again—and this time... it turned out I was pregnant!

Doctors told me: "Without IVF you have no chance of getting pregnant." I thought: "It's never going to happen." The good old-fashioned way worked. It's like being given a gift. I have the joy of being pregnant. It puts the diet in perspective. (Meg, 39)

Nine months later, we got this message:

I had a baby girl in November who was seven pounds and four ounces, nineteen inches, and she had a full head of hair! We're so incredibly ecstatic. (Meg)

About six million men and women of reproductive age in the United States (10 percent) are affected by infertility. Approximately 20 percent of these people suffer from "unexplained infertility," i.e., no underlying cause such as hormone irregularities, tubal obstructions, low sperm count, or other medical problems can be found. It is in this "unexplained" arena of reproduction and infertility that celiac disease appears to play a role.

Meg is only one of many patients with a similar story: some were unable to get pregnant; others kept having miscarriages until celiac disease was diagnosed. Unfortunately, the diagnosis may come too late for those women whose menopause has already arrived—which may explain the studies indicating that people with celiac disease have fewer children.

While the exact magnitude of the problem in the celiac community has not been definitively quantified, studies over the past few years implicated celiac disease as a possible cause of many unexplained fertility cases. Most of these studies were conducted in Europe and South America, where patients attending an infertility clinic will be routinely tested for celiac disease. In the United States, this type of testing would be the exception—celiac disease is off the radar screens of most infertility doctors in this country.

Different European studies have examined both male and female infertility. The studies showed a higher prevalence of unexplained infertility in women.

> *I kept going back to the doctor and saying "Something's wrong."* . . .
> *I lost the baby one week before she was due.* (Nancy, 32)

Celiac disease has been associated with many gynecological, obstetrical, and fertility problems, including:

- Delayed onset of menstruation (menarche)
- Early menopause
- Menstrual irregularities
- Spontaneous miscarriages
- Poorer pregnancy outcome
- Reduced male fertility
- Sexual behavior (e.g., less frequent intercourse)
- Smaller babies
- Higher perinatal mortality
- Shorter duration of breast-feeding

Unfortunately for patients, the relationship between celiac disease, infertility, and reproductive problems is often recognized only retrospectively; many of the symptoms are attributed to other underlying causes. Moreover, fertility problems in celiac disease are poorly understood. Malabsorption and its associated illnesses and effects may be a factor, but they cannot fully explain the complex mechanisms underlying reproductive problems in celiac disease. Autoimmune factors may also play a role.

What Causes Infertility?

Infertility is a multifactorial condition that can be affected by:

- Physical conditions and diseases involving the reproductive organs
- Genetic diseases
- Frequency and timing of ovulation
- Psychological factors
- Illnesses that affect *the processes* of reproduction

Celiac disease falls into this last category.

The Relationship to Celiac Disease: Effect on Females

Studies have demonstrated that women diagnosed with celiac disease are often able to get pregnant, but have an increased rate of spontaneous abortions (miscarriages), accounting for fewer children. And the prevalence of celiac disease in infertile women appears to be higher than that of the general population.

Females with celiac disease tend to have gynecological problems, including a shortened reproductive period—delayed onset of menstruation and premature menopause—and more irregular periods. (Premature menopause is a contributing factor to osteoporosis; for more on this subject, see Chapter 9.)

An Italian study examining sexual behavior in patients with celiac disease showed a reduced rate of intercourse and lower prevalence of individuals satisfied with their sexual life—both of which improved on the gluten-free diet! The study did not delve into the mechanisms behind this finding. However, it can be postulated that the problems arose because the patients felt truly sick for a long period of time. If you are not having sex, you can neither enjoy it nor get pregnant.

The Relationship to Celiac Disease: Effect on Males

Children and adults with celiac disease are often seen with short stature and growth hormone abnormalities. Often referred to as "failure to thrive" in children, these conditions are part of the numerous hormonal changes that affect both sexes. In males, the effect of these abnormalities extends into the arena of fertility. Studies showed reduced male sex hormones and reduced sperm count in men with celiac disease. This appears to have both a hormonal and nutritional basis. The abnormalities are corrected by a gluten-free diet. Another interesting study reported smaller babies and worse outcomes to pregnancies when the father had celiac disease.

The effect of celiac disease on male health goes further than sperm formations and male sex hormones. Men with celiac disease develop more female-predominant diseases, including osteoporosis and other autoimmune conditions.

What Causes Infertility in Celiac Disease?

The actual mechanisms underlying fertility problems in men with celiac disease are not well understood, and few studies are available. The data is slightly more abundant for females, but the mechanisms underlying the problems have not been fully explained.

Nutritional imbalances, specifically vitamins A and E deficiencies, which affect sperm development, can be a possible factor. The malabsorption of micronutrients essential for the metabolism of sex hormones may play a part.

People with celiac disease have immunological as well as nutritional and hormonal abnormalities. The development of tissue resistance may play a role. This is the autoimmune process in which the body mistakes its own tissue for "foreign" matter and develops antibodies that attack it. The body may target androgens, the male sex hormones, or other gonadal tissue in women. As researchers explore the manifestations of tissue resistance in celiac disease—to bone, thyroid, heart—the autoimmune connection in infertility may come into clearer focus.

The Effect of the Gluten-Free Diet

At first it was just depressing. I was mourning my old foods and almost overwhelmed by the diet. When I got pregnant, I said: "This is worth it!" (Meg, 39)

Even though the main mechanism responsible for reduced fertility in celiac disease is currently unknown, early diagnosis and treatment can have a positive effect on mother, father, and potential children. As with Meg, stories abound of successful outcomes after a year or more on the gluten-free diet. It is equally important that pregnant women with celiac disease maintain a strict gluten-free diet. They must also be mindful of the nutritional demands of the growing fetus and maintain a balanced and well-supplemented vitamin and mineral intake throughout the pregnancy and lactation.

Next Steps

Infertility is a highly emotional and often ambiguous medical issue. When couples are then informed that their problem is due to "unexplained infertility," the few available answers may disappear. Fortunately, **we now have enough evidence to show that celiac disease should**

be considered and ruled out in people who suffer from "unexplained" reproductive and fertility problems. The potential for getting pregnant "the good old-fashioned way" and maintaining that pregnancy becomes a viable option for these patients.

The Celiac Disease Center at Columbia is currently working with infertility experts in the United States on a study of the prevalence of celiac disease in their patient populations. It is vital that well-conducted clinical studies are performed that screen a large group of infertile couples for celiac disease. It is only then that the physicians involved in the care of couples trying to get pregnant will understand that the diagnosis of celiac disease should be considered.

People of reproductive age spend an enormous amount of time, money, and energy trying to get pregnant and carry the pregnancy to term. A gluten-free diet may not be the answer for all of them, but for the select few it can mean a great new start.

14

Autoimmune and Other Related Conditions

I'm convinced that if you have one autoimmune disease, you have ten. They like to stick together.

I was born with two broken legs and my eyes hemorrhaged. It was from osteogenesis imperfecta (OGI), brittle bone disease, a genetic illness. Many times I walked around with fractures that were never really diagnosed. I have had approximately sixty-five fractures that they know of. I had been to so many doctors by seventeen that I wanted to stay away from all of them.

From the time I was a child I hated going to the dinner table, my stomach hurt so much. When I was in high school, I started getting horrendous nausea and severe, severe joint pain. I had severe malaise (discomfort). I had always been an active child, but the rashes, bone pain, and malaise kept getting worse and worse, and I would get infections all the time—pneumonia, dental infections, a cut would get infected. My dentist put me in touch with a rheumatologist. He didn't want to jump to conclusions because a lot of the symptoms of osteogenesis imperfecta and lupus overlap each other. But they did the blood tests, and I had lupus.

When you have these kinds of illnesses, it can become your entire life ... overtake you. Seven years ago, I had a bad lupus attack, well I thought it was a lupus attack and I collapsed on the kitchen floor. I woke up three hours later in the ICU, and my dad said: "They don't know what's the matter." My blood counts were so low I had several transfusions.

And my stomach was so bad. I spent eight months vomiting every meal I consumed.

That summer my father died and my brother had a heatstroke and was in a coma. It was very stressful. I dropped seventy pounds in two months. The doctor said: "This has gone on long enough, you're anorexic. You just don't want to eat." You can't argue with these guys either; when they make a diagnosis, that's it. I knew there was something the matter with me, but no one would listen.

A year or two later, I started to lose my hair. It was alopecia areata. Sometimes you can get that as a complication of lupus: mine was not, it was a separate autoimmune disease. I'm lucky, my hair grew back.

So I was blaming the abdominal pain on lupus because you can have stomach involvement and severe pain. And I would wake up every morning, and my hands would be totally numb and so tingly. I would have to run them under warm water to get the feeling back in them. From what I understand celiac disease can affect your central nervous system, give you neuropathies. But again, lupus can do that, too.

I finally met a gastroenterologist and said: "You have to do something." Well, he did a colonoscopy and an endoscopy. He came back and said: "You have celiac disease."

Celiac disease has been one of the hardest things that has affected me . . . maybe because it's the third autoimmune disease.

Autoimmune disease is like a black cloud always hanging over you saying, "Don't try to run too fast because I'm right behind you!"
(Anna, 40)

The manifestations of celiac disease are like the tentacles of an octopus—reaching out and into all the systems of the body. But autoimmune diseases provide the bulk of the illness burden. **While autoimmune disorders affect approximately 3 percent of the general population, they affect 30 percent of those with celiac disease.** Studies show that more than 30 percent of patients diagnosed after the age of twenty—after prolonged exposure to gluten—develop at least one autoimmune disease. And once a patient develops one autoimmune condition, the odds of developing another are greatly increased. Autoimmune diseases also run in families, but different diseases may affect different family members.

Gender issues are particularly interesting for those with celiac disease. In the general population, women are far more likely than men to develop an autoimmune disease (3:1). In the celiac disease community, the risk is the same for men and women.

While there is very good evidence that patients who have celiac disease have a much higher prevalence of other autoimmune disorders than the general population, the mechanism(s) of the association is debated.

What Causes Autoimmune Disease?

Autoimmune disease occurs when the body targets itself—mistaking "self" for "nonself." In other words, the antibodies that protect us from foreign matter see the body's own proteins and tissues as foreign and attack them. The source of the problem in autoimmune disorders is the immune system—the target organ only displays the symptoms. Essentially, autoimmune disease is an immune system with crossed wires, turning on itself.

While the triggering agent in celiac disease—gluten—has been identified, there is no known environmental trigger for any other autoimmune disease. This makes celiac disease unique among the autoimmune diseases.

The causative factors for the development of autoimmune diseases are believed to be a combination of the following:

Genetics

A common genetic predisposition occurs in many people with autoimmune diseases. Most of the genes associated with these conditions are only partially understood. And one gene does not necessarily precipitate any given disease.

The HLA types (see A Genetic Primer—Fitting the Groove, Chapter 6) that are implicated in celiac disease are also found in diabetes, but researchers do not believe they tell the entire story. The HLA mechanism for recognizing "self" and "nonself" somehow turns on itself in the autoimmune reaction. This causes a cascade of events that damages and destroys tissue and organs throughout the body.

Tissue and Organ Autoantibodies

Antibodies are thought to be predictive of a disorder, i.e., if you have antithyroid antibodies, you are at risk for developing thyroid disease. Therefore, patients with autoimmune conditions have antibodies to a specific organ or tissue, or several.

At diagnosis, patients with celiac disease often have a high rate of autoantibodies to other tissues and organs. These include antithyroid antibodies, antipancreas antibodies, and antinuclear antibodies (ANA).

Once on the gluten-free diet, fewer people with celiac disease have these positive antibodies. In one study, children who had antibodies to thyroid and pancreas tissue lost those antibodies while following a gluten-free diet. This suggests that getting diagnosed with celiac disease and going on a gluten-free diet reverses the risk of getting these autoimmune disorders, at least for children.

Celiac Disease

There is some tantalizing evidence that having celiac disease actually disposes people to having the second (or third) autoimmune disorder. The evidence comes from a study demonstrating that the age of diagnosis of celiac disease correlated with the risk of getting the associated autoimmune disorder. That is, children diagnosed with celiac disease before age two developed autoimmune diseases at the same rate as the rest of the general population (about 3 to 5 percent). There was a linear increase in the prevalence of autoimmune diseases with the increasing age of diagnosis of celiac disease up to age twenty, where 30 percent of the individuals in this study had an autoimmune disorder. This is a compelling case for the early diagnosis of celiac disease and an urgent reason to educate the professional community in the symptoms and risks of celiac disease. Other studies have not confirmed that duration of gluten exposure is a significant risk factor for developing autoimmune diseases.

Which Comes First?

Frequently, the associated autoimmune disease is diagnosed first because it is more obviously symptomatic, while the celiac disease remains silent. Nevertheless, it is believed that celiac disease may come first, predisposing individuals to the development of the autoimmune diseases.

Unfortunately, autoimmune disorders are often so well established by the time of diagnosis of celiac disease—with evidence of organ damage, not just the presence of antibodies—that a reversal of the condition is very unlikely. However, there are some cases in which the associated autoimmune disease actually improves after diagnosis of celiac disease. This has been demonstrated in IgA nephropathy, peripheral neuropathy, hypothyroidism, and cardiomyopathy.

The specific autoimmune diseases associated with celiac disease include diabetes (Chapter 12), peripheral neuropathy (Chapter 7), as well as:

- Thyroid disease
- Sjögren's syndrome
- Addison's disease
- Autoimmune liver disease
- Cardiomyopathy
- Alopecia areata
- Lupus
- Rheumatoid arthritis

Thyroid Disease

After my daughter was born, I was always tired and my thyroid stopped working. I was told that both were pretty common after a pregnancy and that the thyroid often returned to normal. In retrospect, those were the first two symptoms of what would be diagnosed as celiac disease eighteen years later. (Anonymous, 45)

The thyroid is a small gland that has a large presence in the body. Thyroid hormones regulate metabolism, influence muscle and bone growth and development, and affect heart and vascular functions. The hormones also play a role in brain function and behavior.

Autoimmune thyroid disease is the most common autoimmune disease seen and is very commonly found in people with celiac disease. There are two forms of the condition.

Hashimoto's Disease, Hypothyroidism

Hashimoto's disease, an autoimmune form of hypothyroidism (an underactive thyroid gland), is the most common. It is usually diagnosed prior to the celiac disease diagnosis and requires treatment with thyroid hormone replacement. Hypothyroidism can be subclinical for many years, but may manifest when the metabolism of the body is stressed, such as during or after a pregnancy or after a traumatic illness. If the thyroid gland is inflamed due to an autoimmune mechanism, it cannot produce enough of the necessary thyroid hormone just when the body has increased demands for it. This results in clinical hypothyroidism.

Many of the symptoms of hypothyroidism mimic those of celiac disease. These include fatigue, depression, muscle cramps, and constipation. Patients may also have unexplained weight gain, an intolerance to cold (without thyroid hormone the body's metabolic rate drops, leaving the body's thermostat below the comfort zone), or dry, thickened skin and scalp.

Treatment for hypothyroidism is straightforward—thyroid hormones in a bottle—but there can be problems with the therapy. Soy has been implicated as a cause of reduced absorption of thyroid hormone replacement therapy. Interestingly, we have seen two patients diagnosed with celiac disease because their endocrinologist could not explain their increasing thyroid hormone requirements to maintain a normal level of the hormone in their bloodstream. Their astute endocrinologist realized that they were malabsorbing the medication.

Conversely, patients with celiac disease may require a reduced level of thyroid hormone replacement after their intestines have healed. (See The Effect of the Gluten-Free Diet, page 158.)

Graves' Disease, Hyperthyroidism

I was on a strict gluten-free diet and could not gain a pound. I think my doctor thought I was cheating on the diet. (Kathy, 42)

Graves' disease, or *thyrotoxicosis* or *hyperthyroidism* (an overactive thyroid gland), often manifests before the celiac disease diagnosis, but also appears afterward. It occurs due to antibodies that increase thyroid function. Treatment for an overactive thyroid is often more complex than that for an underactive gland.

Patients with hyperthyroidism are treated with antithyroid drugs, which lower the secretion of thyroid hormones. Since these drugs can cause an allergic reaction or lower the body's white blood cell count and therefore resistance to infections, they must be closely monitored. If the overheated gland cannot be quieted down, it is sometimes slowed down with radioactive iodine or surgically removed. The overactive metabolic stimulation of the heart may require specific therapy.

Some of the symptoms of hyperthyroidism also mimic celiac disease. These include muscle weakness, irritability, weight loss, and disrupted sleep patterns. Patients typically have other manifestations of an overactive metabolism, including anxiety, heart palpitations, feeling hot, and protruding eyeballs (a classic sign).

Relation to Celiac Disease

The relation between thyroid disease and celiac disease is statistically high, but the underlying mechanisms are less obvious. Both are autoimmune disorders and, therefore, several factors must be considered:

1. Both celiac disease and thyroid disease are common; therefore, it is more likely that they will occur together more frequently.
2. Celiac disease may predispose to all or any autoimmune disease, including thyroid disease.
3. Physicians often test for thyroid disease because they think that it is common.

Management Issues

There are many highly sensitive and specific tests for thyroid function. We recommend that people have their TSH (thyroid-stimulating hormone) levels measured annually. This is a very good measure of thyroid function. It goes up when people are hypothyroid (stimulating the thyroid to produce more hormones), down when they're hyperthyroid (inhibited by the excess thyroid hormones). If levels are not within normal range, the physician can conduct more specific tests for thyroid problems.

We have identified either hyperthyroidism or hypothyroidism in patients who were referred because of their failure to respond to the gluten-free diet.

The Effect of the Gluten-Free Diet

There is evidence that a gluten-free diet can improve hypothyroidism. Several patients who have been on the diet for a number of years report a lowered need for thyroid replacement hormone. This could be due to several different mechanisms. First, as the celiac disease is treated, and the intestine heals, absorption of the medication can improve. A lowered inflammatory response, possibly due to reduced antibody levels, may reduce inflammation in the thyroid gland.

Sjögren's Syndrome

I never thought about saliva until it was gone. I suck these candies and put these drops in my eyes. It's a pain. I tried a (systemic) medicine for the dryness for about a month and stopped because I was always sweating. My father had it. (Lucy, 60)

Sjögren's syndrome is an autoimmune disease in which the glands that produce mucus/moisture in the mucous membranes of the body become inflamed and/or destroyed. These glands include the salivary glands of the mouth, the lachrymal glands of the eye, the pancreas, which has similar tissue, and the glands that release mucus/moisture into other mucous membranes such as in the nose, lungs, and vagina. Sjögren's runs in families and can cause extreme discomfort as well as interfere with digestion, eyesight, and sexual function. Sjögren's affects about two to four million people, most of whom are women.

Often called "dry eye" or "dry mouth" syndrome, the effect on the salivary and lachrymal glands is particularly important. People have less saliva because all the little glands in the gums and the lips are affected. This can interfere with swallowing to the point that patients must constantly drink liquids with their food in order to get it down their throats. Similar glands, the lachrymal glands, that are responsible for tears may be equally affected. Tears protect the eye from infection as well as enable the lid to open and close. Patients complain of dry, scratchy, or "sticky" eye, especially in the morning.

The pancreas has similar tissue, so patients often have an atrophic (with reduced function) pancreas, which may contribute to malabsorption.

The symptoms of Sjögren's have an interesting overlap with those of celiac disease and several other conditions. In addition to the classic dry eye and dry mouth, patients may complain of neuropathies, joint pain, fatigue, and indigestion—all seen in celiac disease. The indigestion may be caused by a lack of pancreatic enzymes, or by celiac disease itself.

Many of the symptoms of Sjögren's are often attributed to other rheumatoid conditions. Women may have dry vagina and painful intercourse, which might be attributed to menopause. The drying of mucous membranes is also a function of aging. In short, the diagnosis of Sjögren's can be as difficult and delayed as that of celiac disease, especially if the symptoms are mild.

There are specific antibodies present in the blood of some—but not all—patients with Sjögren's syndrome. A test performed by an ophthalmologist may detect a lack of normal tears. A biopsy of the mucous membranes of the mouth may be necessary to detect the inflammation and atrophy of the salivary glands.

Treatment is both topical and systemic. Lubricating drops, tear duct blockers that allow secretions to accumulate in the eyes, and/or systemic medications that stimulate saliva and mucus production can all be used. Some patients complain that the oral saliva medications stimulate a systemic sweat gland response that is not altogether desirable. Other therapies are being explored.

Relation to Celiac Disease

Studies show an increased rate of celiac disease among patients with Sjögren's syndrome. Interestingly, Sjögren's carries an increased risk for lymphoma, as does celiac disease.

The Effect of the Gluten-Free Diet

There is no current research on the effect of the gluten-free diet on the course of Sjögren's syndrome.

Addison's Disease

Addison's disease is an autoimmune mediated atrophy of the adrenal glands. These glands play an important, life-maintaining role in the body's response to stress (regulating blood flow, oxygen, and nutrient supply), metabolism, the immune system, cardiovascular function, and sex hormones. Untreated, it can be fatal, since the body cannot fight off the stress of major trauma or infections.

Patients do not produce enough of the adrenal hormones such as *cortisol* and aldosterone. This causes an increase in *adrenocorticotropic hormone (ACTH)*, a hormone that normally stimulates the release of cortisol. ACTH also stimulates melanocytes (hormones that increase skin pigmentation), which results in the classical clinical appearance of darkened skin.

Patients also have weakness and fatigue, combined with high potassium and low sodium levels due to the effects on the kidneys. While there are specific ways of diagnosing Addison's disease—measuring cortisol and ACTH levels—the physician must know to look for the condition, since its symptoms may suggest other more prevalent conditions.

Studies show a close relationship with celiac disease. Interestingly, JFK was believed to have celiac disease, based on his chronic gastrointestinal problems since childhood, severe osteoporosis, and familial Addison's disease.*

The treatment of Addison's disease is cortisone therapy.

Autoimmune Liver Disease

Several autoimmune liver diseases are associated with celiac disease. The best established relation is with primary biliary cirrhosis (PBC). This condition results from an inflammatory process in the liver affecting the bile ducts. PBC eventually leads to cirrhosis of the liver. While PBC is not common, about 90 percent of the patients are women.

Patients have difficulty excreting *bilirubin* (a waste product of red blood cells) and cholesterol. Bile salts that accumulate in the liver (see The Liver, Chapter 1) may contribute to the major complaint of patients with PBC—itching (*pruritus*). Many also become *jaundiced* (develop yellow skin), caused by the retention of bilirubin, which is secreted along with bile pigments that give urine its characteristic yellow color.

PBC is often suspected because of abnormal liver tests discovered when a patient is being tested for another illness. It requires a liver biopsy to be positively diagnosed as well as the presence of specific autoantibodies in the blood.

The relationship between celiac disease and PBC is so strong that patients with PBC are often screened for celiac disease with or without symptoms. There is currently no satisfactory treatment for the condition.

---

* Peter H. Green, M.D. "Was JFK the Victim of an Undiagnosed Disease Common to the Irish?" Invited Op-Ed contribution. History and Historians. History News Network. November 25, 2002. www.hnn.us.

Patients are usually given bile salts to improve liver function. Bile acid-binding resins may relieve itching. Osteoporosis is common in PBC, and the additional presence of celiac disease will aggravate the bone loss. Liver transplantation is the only definitive therapy.

Cardiomyopathy

Cardiomyopathy is an inflammatory disorder of the heart muscle. There are three types of cardiomyopathy—dilated, hypertrophic, and restrictive. The type found in celiac disease is the most common form, dilated (congestive) cardiomyopathy. In this condition, the heart muscle becomes inflamed, weakens, and, as a result, the heart dilates (enlarges). It cannot pump normally, and most patients develop heart failure. Patients also have *arrythmias* (disturbances in the heart's electrical conduction) that may cause palpitations and further impair cardiac function.

There is evidence that the autoimmune reaction against the heart is directed against tissue transglutaminase (tTG) present in the heart. In patients with an associated autoimmune cardiomyopathy, treatment of the celiac disease with a gluten-free diet has been shown to improve cardiac function.

Alopecia Areata

> My son started losing his hair around seven. They thought it was stress at first. He wears a baseball cap everywhere—it's tough, but his friends are pretty good about it. He has a huge collection of hats and has started matching them to his clothes. (Robin, 42)

Alopecia areata is an autoimmune condition in which patchy areas of total hair loss occur. The scalp is most commonly affected, but it can appear on any hair-bearing parts of the body. There is a well-established association with celiac disease. A recent study from Finland found 2 percent of celiac disease patients with the condition.

Alopecia areata is fairly common and affects men and women equally. The condition usually appears first in childhood. The hair follicles are attacked by the immune system, arresting hair growth for months or years. Some people have a few bare patches; others exhibit more dramatic hair loss. The hair may regrow and fall out again. The definitive diagnosis is usually made with a biopsy of the hair root—after ruling out sex hormone abnormalities, thyroid problems, and other diseases that may have caused the hair loss.

The mechanism(s) that cause alopecia areata are not fully understood, but it is considered to be mainly autoimmune. Stress may play a part in triggering some episodes of hair loss, but the disease is not caused by stress alone.

The condition is treated with steroid injections into the scalp, and topical creams. Immunosuppressant therapy with cyclosporins is sometimes used. Biological therapies that may selectively inhibit the immune response in alopecia areata are in development.

There are reports of a gluten-free diet initiating hair growth in some patients. Along with other dermatological diseases such as psoriasis, patients have gone into remission when adhering to the diet. This would indicate a causative role for gluten in the related autoimmune disorder.

Lupus

Lupus, or systemic lupus erythematosus (SLE), is a multisystem disorder in which the immune system is directed against the body's own tissues; it can result in damage to, or destruction of, vital organs.

Its symptoms mimic those of many other autoimmune diseases such as rheumatoid arthritis, multiple sclerosis, and celiac disease, and it is difficult to diagnose. Patients may have extreme fatigue, joint pain, muscle aches, anemia, mouth sores, and depression.

Its relation to celiac disease is controversial—more research needs to be done in this area.

Rheumatoid Arthritis

Rheumatoid arthritis is an autoimmune disorder affecting the joints, resulting in swelling, pain, stiffness, and loss of joint function. It tends to be symmetrical, affecting both sides of the body equally.

The condition is fairly common, affecting about 1 percent of the United States population. The word *arthritis* literally means joint inflammation, and that characterizes the condition.

Its association with celiac disease is not well established, although some patients report both conditions.

There are other illnesses beyond the autoimmune spectrum that have been studied in relation to celiac disease.

Fibromyalgia

Fibromyalgia is a poorly understood condition characterized by symptoms that mimic many other diseases. Like irritable bowel syndrome, it is often diagnosed when no other underlying cause of or cure for the specific symptoms can be found. And a study by one nationwide celiac disease support group indicated that among adults ultimately diagnosed with celiac disease, 9 percent were originally diagnosed with fibromyalgia and 30 percent with IBS.

The symptoms of fibromyalgia include the following:

- Fatigue
- Muscle and joint pains without any specific underlying abnormality
- GI symptoms, including reflux, non-ulcer dyspepsia
- Noncardiac chest pain

Since many patients with celiac disease have muscle aches, joint pains, GI symptoms, and fatigue, it is understandable that those people might get a label of fibromyalgia.

Some patients will consult rheumatologists for rheumatic-type syndromes that can be due to celiac disease. An example is polymyalgia rheumatica, a very well-defined entity in which people have proximal muscle weakness and a very high sedimentation (ESR) rate (an indication of inflammation). (See Inflammation, Chapter 7.) These patients with celiac disease improve on a gluten-free diet. We have seen some patients with celiac disease who have rather vague musculoskeletal symptoms and a very high ESR. On a gluten-free diet, the very high ESR and the symptoms have resolved. This indicates that celiac disease is truly a systemic inflammatory disorder.

The diagnosis of fibromyalgia is difficult to define—it is based on a number of symptoms that can be due to other conditions. And celiac disease is one of them. This is further evidence that different so-called "silent" symptoms need to be taken seriously by physicians and thoroughly evaluated before a diagnosis of fibromyalgia (or IBS) is given.

Aphthous Stomatitis

Aphthous stomatitis is an autoimmune condition in which people get canker sores in their mouth. Some patients have severe cases; others get them intermittently. Many patients report this as one of the key "in retrospect" symptoms from their childhood.

There is a statistical association with celiac disease. Some people get better on a gluten-free diet and have relapses when exposed to gluten.

Multiple Sclerosis (MS)

MS is an autoimmune disease that affects the central nervous system. Myelin, a fatty tissue surrounding and protecting nerve fibers, is damaged or destroyed. It is lost in multiple areas, leaving scar tissue (sclerosis).

Myelin not only protects nerve fibers, but enables the nerves to conduct electrical impulses to and from the brain. The disruption of these impulses produces the various symptoms of MS.

The current studies done on the relation between MS and celiac disease show no increased incidence.

Autism Spectrum Disorder (ASD)

Autism spectrum disorder is characterized by impairments in social communication and restricted and repetitive behaviors. These impairments can range from mild to severe. To date, no studies have shown an association between ASD and celiac disease, even though many children with ASD are placed on a gluten- and casein-free diet as therapy. (Casein is the major protein found in milk.)

Gastrointestinal complaints and conditions are among the most common medical issues associated with ASD. Diarrhea, constipation, and GERD are often reported. This may be a direct effect of certain behaviors ("holding it in" may result in constipation), or the GI complaint may affect their behavior as well as their physical well-being.

Many nonverbal children who cannot simply say that their tummies hurt express distress in other ways. A child in pain may withdraw or engage in self-injurious behavior (i.e., bite himself or herself) or have a tantrum in order to get attention so that someone will come to help. This does not mean that all children who display disruptive behaviors are masking GI symptoms; and GI issues are not seen as a singular problem in ASD—a subset of typical children also have GI issues—but GI symptoms may be an extra barrier to ameliorating symptoms and effecting treatment.

Individuals with GI issues and ASD need to be diagnosed and treated by a gastroenterologist in order to isolate and properly treat their symptoms.

The role of gluten in the development, progress, and treatment of ASD is complex and under intense scrutiny in different settings. It is possible that the presence of IgG antigliadin antibodies may indicate a subset of children who may benefit from a gluten-free diet.

Studies have shown that there are increased food antibodies (IgG antigliadin antibodies and anticasein antibodies) in a subset of children with autism who have GI symptoms. These are non-celiac antibodies. While this suggests a gut-brain interaction, we do not know the direction of this interaction (i.e., is the brain affecting gut permeability or vice versa?). The presence of antibodies has to be shown to have a direct effect on brain function or dysfunction if it is to have scientific significance as a causative factor. Nevertheless, this immune response may help to identify novel biomarkers of ASD and offer new insights into the disease mechanisms for some of those with ASD.

But these antibodies must be studied further to determine when they develop and how they relate to the child's development. We must be careful not to confuse association with cause.

Gastrointestinal dysfunction may provide a window to better understanding both autism and the brain in autism. It is a bidirectional avenue that may hold answers even in those without GI disorders. Potentially it could mean that a drug targeting the intestines might help neuropsychiatric conditions.

Pitfalls of a Gluten-Free Diet for ASD

There are many feeding issues in children with ASD. They are more "picky" eaters than those in the general population, perhaps as a manifestation of restricted and repetitive behaviors that are a hallmark of the disorder. The gluten-free diet is often low in fiber and essential nutrients, and this may only compound the problem. Recent studies on the presence of heavy metals in people on a gluten-free diet raise possible neurological complications that need to be studied further.

Therefore, parents should be aware that they are adding nutritional as well as food choice limitations to a population already burdened by restrictions.

The use of gluten-free and/or casein-free diets in people with ASD is controversial. Scientific studies have not proved that there are objective changes in behaviors in children on these diets.

Attention-Deficit/Hyperactivity Disorder (ADHD)

The range of developmental disorders in children is extremely diverse. It includes attention and memory problems, hyperactivity, childhood depression (see Chapter 10), underachievement, and disruptive behavior. The link between gluten and behavioral problems in children with celiac disease is well documented in the scientific literature. The association is demonstrated by the many children who are treated at the Center with histories of psychological problems and cognitive disorders that improve on a gluten-free diet.

We undertook a long-term study with a group of children attending an ADHD clinic to determine whether there was an increased prevalence of celiac disease. Most intriguingly, while none of the children had celiac disease, all of the children had high levels of antigliadin antibodies. This supports recent studies showing that non-celiac gluten sensitivity can present outside of the intestine and often involves the nervous system. (See Chapter 7.)

We believe that future research will reinforce the link between food and cognitive developmental disorders, with celiac disease and non-celiac gluten sensitivity as a major bridge between these problems.

Schizophrenia

Schizophrenia affects about 1 percent of the population. Its association with celiac disease has been the subject of several studies over the past few years. While some of the studies have found no increased prevalence, several more recent ones have shown an almost twofold increase in celiac disease in schizophrenic patients. A percentage of these patients also have non-celiac gluten sensitivity manifested by antigliadin antibodies. This connection raises the question of the relation between celiac disease and a variety of psychiatric disorders.

As we wrote about in *Gluten Exposed* (2017) the association of bread with madness dates back to the Middle Ages, when rye was susceptible to ergot, a fungus containing chemicals that resemble LSD. When eaten, it caused convulsions, pain, and a type of "madness" called St. Anthony's Fire, or ergot poisoning. The "madness" symptoms were then attached to schizophrenia. In the 1920s, the "intestinal intoxication" theory of schizophrenia was popular. Papers in the 1960s referred to schizophrenia as "bread madness."

While the specific causes of schizophrenia are unknown, contributing factors appear to include a genetic predisposition interacting with complex environmental and neurotransmitter disturbances.

A Danish population study found an association between schizophrenia and a larger range of autoimmune diseases. A common genetic susceptibility, autoantibodies, and the genetic role in intestinal permeability have been suggested as possible causes.

Larger studies are needed to confirm the association between gluten and schizophrenia—the so-called bread madness—and to examine the underlying mechanisms by which this occurs.

Dental Enamel Defects

Dental enamel defects are very common in patients with celiac disease. They consist of imperfections in the teeth affecting the enamel, or outer surface, of the tooth. They may manifest as white or brown spots on the tooth, or, in severe forms, ridges and malformed teeth. The defects are symmetrical and bilateral (found on both sides).

Several studies from Europe indicate that patients with celiac disease have a higher incidence of dental enamel defects than non-celiacs. The damage to the teeth occurs if celiac disease is present as the teeth are forming. Patients often have teeth laminated or capped because of imperfect-appearing teeth—covering up what may be an indication of celiac disease.

Dr. Theologos Ted Malahias, D.D.S., a dentist studying these defects with us, feels that they are "another piece of the puzzle." He explains that "the mouth is a mirror of your health." Aphthous ulcers (canker sores), whose frequency of occurrence decreases with the start of a gluten-free diet, may also be an indication of celiac disease.

Nutritional deficiencies, or immunological processes during infancy (such as celiac disease), infections in childhood (such as chicken pox, scarlet fever, rubella), and excess fluoride while the teeth are forming can also cause enamel defects.

A patient diagnosed with celiac disease should look for dental enamel defects and frequent aphthous ulcers in first- and second-degree relatives, especially those who appear to be asymptomatic. Because of the risk of gluten ingestion, you should inform your dentist of your celiac disease diagnosis to ensure that all polishing pastes, fluoride, and prescribed medications are gluten-free.

Hopefully, dentists encountering a patient with bilateral and symmetrical dental enamel defects will add celiac disease to the list of possible causes, especially when there is a medical history suggestive of celiac disease, or if the patient has a first-degree relative with the condition.

Raynaud's Syndrome

A number of patients with celiac disease also have Raynaud's syndrome, a circulatory condition whose underlying cause is unknown. It is regarded as a connective tissue disorder. It is not believed to be inherited, but it is frequently seen in multiple family members.

Raynaud's is caused by an inappropriate, extreme constriction of the blood vessels in the extremities of the body (hands, fingers, feet, toes) due to cold temperatures. On exposure to cold, the small arteries in the extremities constrict (close), and the affected part becomes pale and often blue and returns to normal color on warming. People with Raynaud's complain of cold hands or feet.

A single study showed that it was not more common in people with celiac disease than in the general population.

Genetic Disorders

Certain genetically determined syndromes have a higher rate of celiac disease than that of the general population. These include:

- Down syndrome
- Turner syndrome
- Williams syndrome
- IgA deficiency

The presence of some of these disorders can complicate blood tests for celiac disease, in particular IgA deficiency. (See Blood Tests, Chapter 4.)

The prevalence with Down patients is particularly high. These people used to die very young because they are susceptible to many different illnesses, including different malignancies and congenital heart disease. Now, with improved cardiac surgery and better care, they are living longer and consequently getting many associated disorders.

People with Down may not be able to report symptoms as well as other individuals. As a result, it is advised that they be screened for thyroid dysfunction and celiac disease. Screening is also recommended for other genetic disorders, as it decreases the likelihood of getting complications and may improve the response to other treatments.

A Final Word

The autoimmune connection is particularly strong in the celiac disease community. While approximately 10 percent of first-degree relatives have celiac disease, the figure skyrockets if relatives have an autoimmune disease. **The relative with an autoimmune disease has up to a 25 percent chance of having celiac disease.**

When a patient has, or develops, another autoimmune or related disorder, the condition must be treated independently. Many patients with celiac disease talk about "collecting doctors" for their various symptoms and illnesses. It is important that each of them understands the celiac disease connection to their specialty.

Of all the autoimmune disorders, the most well-established relationships with celiac disease are (in no particular order):

- Type 1, IDDM (insulin-dependent diabetes mellitus)
- Peripheral neuropathy
- Thyroiditis
- Primary biliary cirrhosis
- Sjögren's syndrome
- Aphthous stomatitis
- Cardiomyopathy
- Addison's disease

While we cannot change the genes that may predispose us to these conditions, we can eliminate gluten from our diets and quiet the inflammatory and immune responses that have been indicated as factors in most of these diseases.

Unfortunately, while the early diagnosis of celiac disease may avert the manifestation of these diseases, once they affect specific organs and tissues, much of the damage may have already occurred. A gluten-free diet may be beneficial in some cases, but it will not necessarily cure other related conditions once they are well established. To get it right, it is important to get it early.

PART III

UNDERSTANDING AND TREATING CELIAC DISEASE

MEDICAL MANAGEMENT

Healing is a matter of time, but it is sometimes also a matter of opportunity.

—Hippocrates, *Precepts*

15

What You Need to Know— and Do—After Diagnosis

The doctor said: "You have celiac disease; go find someone to talk to about the diet you'll be on for the rest of your life . . ." and that was it! (Ed, 45)

After diagnosis, it is not uncommon for patients to be given dietary counseling by their doctor that consists of: "Go to the Internet and find out what to eat, come back if you need to. Good luck." These doctors still assume that celiac disease is a straightforward food-related condition that will "clear up" when gluten disappears from the diet.

Many patients suffer from one or more of the related conditions described in the previous chapters and suddenly feel overwhelmed and/ or abandoned. The parents of small children who are still very sick or malnourished must immediately cope with crucial medical and developmental aspects, as well as nutritional issues. Dietary advice is critical, and the first step in managing the condition must start at the doctor's office.

Treating the Patient, Not the Refrigerator

Celiac disease is a lifelong, serious medical condition that can take time and energy to master. Even if a patient looks and feels well, many encounter medical and nutritional complications along the way. Celiac disease, like diabetes, has long-term consequences and manifestations that need to be understood and treated.

It is obvious that treatment after diagnosis is based on the severity of your condition when diagnosed. The patient with severe symptoms or ancillary autoimmune diseases will normally seek out and receive continuing medical care. Asymptomatic patients sometimes question the diagnosis and the need for a strict gluten-free diet, let alone any medical follow-up. But every patient with celiac disease needs a certain level of care in order to regain strength and remain healthy. The following should be considered a standard checklist for *all* newly diagnosed patients.

Dietary Counseling About the Gluten-Free Diet

Patients told to go on a gluten-free diet need to consult with a registered dietician who is aware of celiac disease in order to learn the basics as well as subtleties of the diet. The role of the dietician is to ensure that every person with celiac disease has a balanced, healthy, and varied gluten-free diet that does not simply consist of eating the same "safe" products over and over again. Nutritionists can be found through university celiac disease centers, support groups, referring physicians, and the Academy of Nutrition and Dietetics.

There is a great deal of medical and nutritional information on the Internet. Patients must approach this information with *care and caution,* as it also contains a great deal of misinformation. Many sites do not state how often they are updated, or whether they have actual medical personnel who are experts in the disease regularly reviewing content.

Assessment of Nutritional Deficiencies

Every patient with celiac disease needs *nutritional* counseling, as well as *dietary* counseling. Whether symptoms have been dramatic or mild, vitamin deficiencies need to be explored and treated.

Despite the small intestine's amazing ability to compensate for damage to the villi, long-term malabsorption of even small amounts of iron, folic acid, and vitamin B_{12} can impact the body's ability to function properly. Blood levels of these nutrients, as well as calcium, vitamin D, copper, and zinc, should be measured, and if levels are low enough, supplements may be appropriate. (Vitamin B_{12} is given by injection.) If bone density is depleted to the point of osteopenia or osteoporosis, calcium supplements may be warranted to augment dietary intake.

Vitamins and minerals are most efficiently absorbed through a balanced diet. Despite their current popularity, the long-term benefits of multivitamin and mineral supplements to "bolster" the body have not been scientifically studied or assessed for people with celiac disease. In fact, they may be harmful in large amounts. Furthermore, it is also difficult to find science behind the claims of most dietary supplements, and many contain hidden gluten. (See Chapter 23.) For most patients, vitamin and/or mineral supplements are indicated only when they are depleted through disease, or when the patient is not able to consume a healthy balanced diet.

Unfortunately, some patients with classic, severe celiac disease may have profound weight loss and malabsorption syndrome. These patients can be extremely nutritionally depleted due to extended illness prior to diagnosis. Some patients need to be admitted to the hospital for *parenteral* (intravenous) nutrition that bypasses the injured bowel and is delivered directly into the bloodstream.

Some patients may also be severely anemic due to iron, folate, or vitamin B_{12} deficiency and may even require a blood transfusion. Although it is very rare, some people need steroids to suppress the inflammation caused by the disease long enough for the gluten-free diet to begin to work.

Patients who are very ill should eat a few safe and simple foods. This may include rice, baked potatoes, meat without condiments, and cooked vegetables. These people may initially find it prudent to avoid consuming commercially prepared food as well as eating out at restaurants. They can gradually diversify their diet as their symptoms abate and their knowledge base about a gluten-free diet increases.

Medication Assessment

Many people take medications regularly—as frequently as two to three times a day—and it is important that they are gluten-free. This includes **all prescription drugs, over-the-counter medications, vitamins, and supplements.** Vitamins and supplements are all too often the "hidden" problem in nonresponsive celiac disease. It is important to assess all "inactive" ingredients in a medication or supplement because it may contain binders or suspensions with gluten.

Bone Density Determination

Osteoporosis is a silent disease that is often only discovered after it becomes severe enough to cause a fall or broken bone. Since years of calcium malabsorption may make bones porous or brittle, it is commonly found in patients with celiac disease. Men should also be tested for bone density; they tend to have more severe osteoporosis than women with celiac disease.

Adult patients should have a bone density test and, if osteoporosis or osteopenia is present, should have their parathyroid hormone, calcium, and vitamin D levels measured. This will rule out potential underlying calcium malabsorption that may impact and determine the proper course of therapy.

Pneumococcal Vaccination

Patients with celiac disease are initially more susceptible to pneumococcal pneumonia. This is due to the fact that *hyposplenism,* or an inadequately functioning spleen, is common in active celiac disease, and the spleen is important in fighting bacterial infections caused by pneumococcal bacteria. While a pneumococcal vaccination is recommended in the general population for individuals over the age of fifty, it should be considered for any adult with celiac disease. It is usually repeated every five years. Guidelines for children are not established and should be discussed with their celiac disease doctor.

It is a common misconception that patients with celiac disease are immunocompromised or more prone than the rest of the population to infections. This is not medically accurate. The immune system is not compromised; it is in fact *overactive.* Patients with celiac disease are only at risk for conditions based on specific encapsulated organisms such as pneumococcal pneumonia or meningococcal infections that require the spleen to combat them.

Screening of Family Members

Celiac disease is a genetic condition. It is advisable to screen all first-degree relatives because early diagnosis can prevent the development of associated autoimmune diseases, osteoporosis, and symptomatic celiac disease.

There is nothing to gain—and much to lose—by ignoring the genetic predisposition. Celiac disease should be caught early, before complications can set in. (For more, see Chapter 17.)

Monitoring of Blood Antibody Levels

Patients with moderate to severe symptoms should have follow-up antibody levels measured at six to twelve months. All patients should have follow-up blood work after a year on the gluten-free diet. While most patients have normal levels by that time, some individuals may take much longer to normalize.

Many parents are anxious to retest sick children as soon as possible. Tests performed before the gut has had time to normalize will only unnecessarily increase that anxiety. Unless a child—or adult—shows no clinical improvement on the diet or symptoms increase, waiting for four to six months before repeating the blood tests is advised.

Repeat of Biopsy

Normalization of antibody levels does not indicate the gut mucosa has healed. While there is no specific agreement between experts, a repeat biopsy is often performed to assess a patient's response to the diet. However, a repeat biopsy early in the course of the diet may not show sufficient improvement. We recommend a follow-up biopsy at about two to three years to assess optimal improvement.

Patients who are not doing well on the diet, due to persistent abdominal complaints or diarrhea, may need to undergo earlier or more frequent endoscopy and biopsy to assess the status of the celiac disease. In these cases, the biopsy is used to determine whether there are other complicating conditions. (See Chapter 16.)

While many patients will have normal biopsies during follow-up procedures, some patients have persistent villous atrophy. Some older patients will never show complete healing. The persistent villous atrophy may be due to ongoing gluten ingestion, whether inadvertent or conscious. In this situation, compliance with the diet may need to be addressed by a dietician to determine the source of potential gluten ingestion. If the biopsy continues to show inflammation, the immune system is being continually challenged and the long-term effects may be damaging to other systems in the body.

Screening for Malignancies

Patients with celiac disease are at an increased risk for the development of some specific types of malignancies. (See Chapter 8.) Adults need to attend to this aspect of their health care and have routine screenings. The good news is that after following a gluten-free diet for five years, the malignancy rates in most studies fall to that of the general population.

An adequate yearly physical exam that includes palpating lymph nodes, a breast exam, and a rectal exam looking for blood is recommended. A colonoscopy should be scheduled for patients starting at fifty. It should be performed at an earlier age if there is a family history of adenocarcinoma or blood occurs in the stool.

General Health Measures

Watch Your Weight and Your Cholesterol

Weight loss after starting the diet is not uncommon. Many patients are afraid of eating the wrong foods and actually decrease their caloric intake. However, patients starting a gluten-free diet need to be aware that they are at an increased risk for weight gain and elevated cholesterol levels once on the diet. While the causes of the latter are not clear-cut, one factor is the more efficient absorption of food (including fats) once the inflamed intestine is treated with a gluten-free diet. And many gluten-free treats may be higher in fat.

> I remember my whole life was trying to gain weight. My New Year's resolution was: I'm going to try to gain five pounds this year. So I was hungry all the time, as many newly diagnosed celiacs are, and I would weigh myself every day. And every day I was gaining a half a pound . . . and then I started to calculate what that would mean at the end of the year. . . . So when I reached the weight I thought I should be, I decided to stop all the feeding. (Susan)

Many patients who have been underweight for years start to gain weight and just keep going. For those patients who are already overweight when diagnosed, this will obviously become a greater problem.

Patients whose cholesterol rises because of dietary changes and/or improved absorption should be monitored and treated appropriately by diet and, if necessary, with medications.

Have a Yearly Physical and Celiac-Specific Evaluation

Patients with diabetes normally see their diabetologist several times a year. Similarly, those with high blood pressure are checked regularly. Patients with celiac disease should have a similar mind-set—they have a chronic condition that requires monitoring. They need to have their GI tract checked as well as any other autoimmune condition that they may have acquired as part of the celiac disease spectrum. While noninvasive tests of the small intestine are not very sensitive, patients with celiac disease should have annual physical examinations as well as fecal testing for blood in the stool.

In addition to the blood work normally ordered by their physicians, patients with celiac disease should have a yearly celiac antibody test, as well as tests to determine that their calcium, iron, vitamin, and thyroid function levels are normal. It is important that a more extensive evaluation of vitamin and mineral status be done if patients are not taking vitamin or mineral supplements. Nutritional deficiencies are common in those with celiac disease on a gluten-free diet.

Other evaluations may be necessary if new symptoms develop. Numbness or tingling in fingers or toes may indicate neurological involvement, and copper, vitamin B_6, and vitamin E levels should be checked. If bone density has not improved—or has gotten worse—vitamin D and parathyroid status need to be reassessed.

Medical management is the first important component in treating celiac disease. For some with mild or silent manifestations, it may appear unnecessary. After being on the diet for a while, many patients feel that (1) they know more than the health care provider (and some do!), and (2) treatment stops at the end of their fork. In fact, the need for adequate medical follow-up was one of the recommendations of the NIH Consensus Conference. It is a crucial step in controlling the symptoms and long-term complications of the disease and preventing further illness.

MEDICAL CHECKLIST

___ Dietary counseling

___ Assess nutritional deficiencies

___ Medication assessment

___ Bone density assessment

___ Pneumococcal vaccination (every 5 years)

___ Shingles vaccination

___ Screen family members

___ Follow-up blood antibody levels (yearly)

___ Repeat biopsy

___ Malignancy screening at appropriate ages

___ Weight and cholesterol assessment

___ Yearly physical and celiac evaluation

16

Why Symptoms Persist—
I'm on the Diet and Not
Getting Better

My energy level is better, but I still get stomachaches and diarrhea.
(Cindy, 45)

A gluten-free diet can have a magical effect on the mind and body of a patient who has suffered for months, sometimes years, with symptoms and complaints. Stories abound of joints that stop aching, headaches that become less frequent, mental and mood clouds that lift, stomachaches that disappear. The bathroom is no longer the most visited room in the house. In children, the response can be immediate and dramatic.

Not everyone gets well rapidly. Some patients are simply slow responders and require months (or more) to see an improvement. Medically, the time frame hinges on the nature, severity, and duration of symptoms prior to diagnosis. It is also impacted by the number of ancillary conditions that may complicate the process.

The main reasons why symptoms persist, or even worsen, once on a gluten-free diet include:

1. You are still getting gluten. This is the major cause of a poor response to the diet. It is not unusual for patients to inadvertently consume gluten. Classic examples are regularly ingested communion wafers, a prescribed medication, or a vitamin or dietary supplement.

Your diet is only as good as the information it is based upon. You may be strictly on the wrong diet. Eating "Corn" Flakes or "Rice" Krispies for breakfast is fine, but not if they have malt from barley added as a sweetener.

2. The ongoing inflammatory process. A key component in the healing process is the residual effect of the inflammatory process involved in the disease. All of the cells in the immune arsenal (see Chapter 2) have their own half-life (or lifetime of activity). So the inflammatory process will continue for a period of time even if you arrest the initiating factor (i.e., gluten).

3. You have a common associated condition that also requires treatment. These include lactose or fructose intolerance, pancreatic insufficiency, bacterial overgrowth, or microscopic colitis.

4. There is something else medically wrong. Patients may be intolerant of other foods, have irritable bowel syndrome, inflammatory bowel disease, ulcerative jejunitis, lymphoma, or Addison's disease, to name a few.

5. You have true refractory celiac disease. (See explanation, page 185.) Rare, but possible.

6. You were given the wrong diagnosis and do not have celiac disease. It is impossible to get better on the wrong therapy. This occurs most often when the diagnosis is not well established initially. Blood and biopsy tests may need to be reviewed.

If dietary compliance is good and the diagnosis is correct, it may be necessary to explore specific associated conditions as the potential cause of continued symptoms. These conditions may exist as part of the celiac disease spectrum or as totally separate medical diagnoses.

Lactose Intolerance

Lactose is the carbohydrate in milk that is digested in the small intestine by the enzyme lactase. If lactose is not digested and absorbed, it remains in the chyme and the sugars are broken down by bacteria when it reaches the colon. This produces gas and bloating and diarrhea. (See Intestinal Problems, Chapter 3.)

Primary lactose intolerance is a genetic lack of lactase, which is normally present in the brush border of the small intestine. It is a normal, genetically programmed disorder that occurs in about 25 percent of the U.S. population, more so in certain ethnic groups. Secondary lactose intolerance occurs as a result of any disease that damages or destroys the brush border, such as celiac disease. It can also occur as a result of parasites or viral infections.

People with primary lactose intolerance can take pills with lactase when eating milk or milk products. Secondary lactose intolerance can also be treated with lactase, but usually disappears once the intestine heals and enzyme production returns to normal.

Pancreatic Insufficiency

The doctor put me on pancreatic enzymes—it helped so much with the diarrhea. (Abel, 41)

The pancreas is an organ that has two simultaneous functions. It is an endocrine gland that secretes hormones (e.g., insulin, glucagon) that regulate carbohydrate metabolism and maintain blood sugar at optimal levels. Concurrently, it acts as an *exocrine* gland that secretes enzymes (e.g., trypsin, lipase, amylase) that are necessary for the digestion of specific foods. This exocrine function is dependent on stimulation from the GI tract. (See Chapter 1.)

Pancreatic enzymes are released in response to hormones secreted from the stomach (e.g., gastrin) and small intestine (e.g., secretin, CCK). These hormone "messengers" are triggered by the arrival of food in these sections of the digestive tract. When these hormones are not properly produced in the intestinal tract due to villous atrophy in celiac disease, the pancreas may not receive the stimulus it needs to function properly.

This insufficiency is treated with enzyme replacement to reverse the effect. As the intestine recovers, it starts to produce hormones normally and the body can produce its own pancreatic enzymes. In fact, a patient would have to lose more than 50 percent of pancreatic function to have malabsorption.

Chronic pancreatitis is another disease process. It is a chronic inflammatory condition that can cause *fibrosis* (scarring) and atrophy of the exocrine glands. Some people benefit from long-term pancreatic enzyme replacement.

Bacterial Overgrowth

Bacterial overgrowth is another cause of continuing symptoms. It is defined as the contamination of the small intestine by bacteria that are usually inhabitants of the colon. The small intestine is usually not contaminated by bacteria because it is regularly bathed in and disinfected by a complement of acids, enzymes, and antibodies. Their actions rid it of most foreign bacteria. This process is aided by the constant peristaltic activity of the small intestine. When any one or many of these mechanisms are damaged, the usual defenses that protect the small intestine break down and bacterial overgrowth can occur.

Patients with celiac disease who routinely take antacids or anti-acid-secreting drugs are at added risk for bacterial overgrowth because the protective effort of stomach acid is decreased.

Bacterial overgrowth is easily diagnosed by the use of a breath test (see Chapter 4) and is effectively treated with antibiotics. The condition normally responds to a single dose of antibiotics, but may require rotating antibiotics to keep the bowel free of contamination. Many people with celiac disease who continue to have symptoms respond to Pepto-Bismol. This is probably because of its antibacterial effect.

Once people are on a gluten-free diet and begin to get better, their intestinal motility returns, enzyme and antibody production return to normal, and the body uses its normal mechanisms to prevent bacterial overgrowth.

Microscopic Colitis

I would eat food and it would run through me—it was like water. I couldn't hold on to anything—like an intestinal collapse. There was no way of stopping it. I was disappearing. (Laura, 43)

Microscopic colitis—also called lymphocytic colitis or collagenous colitis—is an autoimmune condition in which the colon becomes inflamed. It has a strong association with celiac disease, typically where symptoms persist while on a gluten-free diet, but is a separate autoimmune condition.

Microscopic colitis is characterized by a specific form of inflammation in the colon and watery diarrhea, with no underlying infection or inflammatory bowel disease. There is a tremendous range of severity in the disease, but, unlike with other forms of colitis, the colon looks normal during colonoscopy and requires a biopsy for diagnosis. It appears in conditions other than celiac disease, but people diagnosed with microscopic colitis often are screened for celiac disease.

Microscopic colitis is not a very common condition, and there have not been many studies on effective treatment. Some over-the-counter drugs may be beneficial, such as Pepto-Bismol and Metamucil. Some patients require immunosuppressive drugs.

Refractory Celiac Disease

I've been really good about the diet—I watch everything I eat. I do eat out a lot, but only where I know I'm safe.... But my last biopsy was still totally flat. I don't know what I'm doing wrong or what more I can do. Maybe stop eating. (Anonymous, 50)

Primary refractory celiac disease (RCD I) is the term used for patients with celiac disease who have ongoing symptoms of malabsorption and persistent villous atrophy after going on a gluten-free diet for at least six months and in whom pancreatic insufficiency, bacterial overgrowth, microscopic colitis, and small intestinal lymphoma have been ruled out. This is mainly a diagnosis of exclusion. It is *not* just the persistence of villous atrophy in a patient who is otherwise doing well with the diet.

Some patients initially appear to do extremely well on the diet and then relapse despite compliance. This is secondary refractory celiac disease (RCD II) and extremely rare. Treatments are lacking but results are promising on the trial of an anti-IL15 antibody. Steroids are the mainstay of treatment. In these patients, refractory celiac disease develops during the course of celiac disease. Studies have been done to determine whether these patients actually have celiac disease. In terms of pathology, both conditions are similar.

Refractory celiac disease can have serious consequences—one is malignancy. Some patients with refractory celiac disease have abnormal lymphocytes (white blood cells), called *clonal lymphocytes,* that are similar to those seen in people with lymphoma. Patients with refractory celiac disease are also seen without clonal proliferation. If clonal lymphocytes are present, patients may progress to lymphoma.

Patients with refractory celiac disease may need hospitalization and treatment with intravenous fluids and nutrients as well as antidiarrheal agents.

After eliminating any other possible reason for the condition—double-checking the diagnosis, ruling out dietary indiscretion and bacterial overgrowth, and using pancreatic supplements—drugs such as cyclosporins and azathioprine (Imuran) are used as treatment for patients with refractory celiac disease. They have fewer side effects than steroids.

Steroid Therapy

Steroid hormones are produced by the adrenal glands and have a profound effect on protein synthesis and cellular activity in the body. They are used therapeutically in severe or refractory cases of celiac disease to stop the immune reaction and inflammation and to promote the healing of the intestine. Although steroids have been routinely prescribed for inflammatory bowel disease and other illnesses since the 1940s, most physicians are hesitant to use them because of side effects.

Steroid therapy puts patients at risk for:

- Infections
- Bone problems (both osteoporosis and avascular necrosis, where round bones such as the hip, heel, knee, and shoulder lose their blood supply and deteriorate, sometimes requiring replacement)
- Diabetes
- Cosmetic effects (continued use can cause facial rounding, hirsutism, a buffalo hump, and severe swelling)

The duration of steroid therapy varies. Patients with true refractory celiac disease with clonal lymphocytes (see page 185) may remain on the drugs indefinitely. Without that, patients stay on the steroids only long enough to give their intestines a chance to recover.

Skin Manifestations

Patients with dermatitis herpetiformis may not respond rapidly to a gluten-free diet. This may be a result of sensitivity to iodides or nonsteroidal anti-inflammatory drugs (NSAIDs) such as aspirin or ibuprofen, or the fact that the IgA deposits in the skin respond more slowly to the removal of gluten from the system. This slow response should not be construed as a nonresponse. Patients with dermatitis herpetiformis must often be more patient patients.

Forms of Gluten Ingestion

There are in reality two forms of gluten ingestion. There is *chronic* exposure that results in the persistence of villous atrophy. In these people the mucosa does not heal and they may or may not have persistent elevated antibodies. This may be intentional or unintentional (due to contamination of a regularly consumed gluten-free food or medication).

The second common mode is *intermittent* exposure that causes symptoms such as nausea and vomiting but not diarrhea or bloating. If people get intermittent fatigue or bloating it is probably not gluten but something else you are eating, possibly FODMAPs.

FODMAPs

Carbohydrates supply most of the fuel for the body. But, for some people, they also supply much of the gas, bloating, and diarrhea that can be confused with celiac disease.

All carbohydrates are sugars (saccharides) and are found in grains, fibers, fruits, vegetables, plants, roots, and nuts. They are also added by manufacturers to sweeten processed products in a condensed form (e.g., dextrose, corn syrups/fructose, malt, glucose).

FODMAP is the acronym for:

Fermentable

Oligosaccharides—fructans and galacto-oligosaccharides, including wheat, onions and garlic, beans, lentils, and chickpeas

Disaccharides—lactose

Monosaccharides—fructose, including all fruits, high-fructose corn syrup, some vegetables, and grains

And

Polyols—sorbitol, mannitol, xylitol, and maltitol, including the sugar alcohols often used in "sugar-free" products (gums, mints, candies)

While most of the food we eat is broken down and digested in the small intestine, some sugars and insoluble fibers arrive in the large intestine mostly undigested. The bacteria living there dine on them in a process called fermentation. This produces, as a by-product, a large amount of gas and liquid, and triggers symptoms that may cause some people to believe they are getting gluten.

It should be noted that gluten is a fructan (an oligosaccharide or complex carbohydrate) but for many people, the main offender is often onion, garlic, or fructose.

People with celiac disease may also be intolerant to a number of FODMAPs and may need to eliminate them to fully resolve their symptoms. Breath tests can isolate an intolerance to fructose or lactose and help people avoid a full elimination diet to determine which food or foods are the problem.

A FODMAP diet has been created that helps people to avoid the particular sugars that trigger their symptoms. It essentially removes the food supply for the bacteria in the colon that are creating the liquid, gas, and bloating. A FODMAP program is best started under the guidance of a registered dietician or knowledgeable nutritionist.

How Soon Will I Get Better?

After seeking answers for what may be years, most patients want immediate results from the diagnosis. Doctors have no crystal ball answers for the constant query of patients: "When will I get better?" They can observe the actual healing curve in follow-up testing, but they cannot predict its course or outcome. For most, persistent symptoms disappear with proper care and attention. But the medical management of ancillary conditions and complicating factors may be necessary for some patients for months, if not years, after diagnosis. Each patient history is slightly different and contains its own time line and resolution.

17

Follow-Up Testing

My daughter had positive antibodies, but a negative biopsy. What do I do now? (Ron, 37)

We have worked so hard on the diet—going crazy—but the blood tests are still positive! (Beth, 30)

Nothing in medicine is 100 percent. While a diagnosis of celiac disease gives most patients the solution they have been seeking, for others the diagnostic tests are more suggestive than definitive. This leaves the doctor with various alternatives—and many patients with inadequate answers. After years of symptoms, most patients want resolution: "Do I have this disease or don't I?"

Some patients do not respond or heal as rapidly as they hoped and question either the diagnosis or treatment.

Another problem may arise when a diagnosed patient enthusiastically seeks out the genetic components of celiac disease. Family members may suddenly find themselves the object of unwanted attention—the new patients are pointing a finger and diagnosing celiac disease in their relatives.

Follow-up testing can play an important role in all of these pictures. It helps to:

- Reexamine false negative and false positive diagnostic tests
- Determine the ongoing medical management of celiac disease
- Determine potential complications and suggest preventative therapy necessary for patients as well as their families

These tests range from blood tests and repeat biopsies to genetic screening and capsule endoscopies (patients swallow a miniature camera that takes pictures as it traverses the digestive tract). For patients with multiple symptoms, these tests help to capture the spectrum of celiac disease in order to treat it more effectively. In many families, it exposes more of the celiac iceberg.

Follow-Up Blood Tests

After six to twelve months on a gluten-free diet, follow-up antibody blood tests are usually negative. They are a reasonable way to assess compliance to the diet. A typical problem arises when patients have blood work done too soon and/or too often. It is necessary to give the body time to respond to the gluten-free diet, even in small children who typically heal and respond faster.

If the blood tests never become negative, there is a serious question of whether the patient is on a gluten-free diet. Patients should expect a definite trend down, even if it takes a year or more to become negative. Minor dietary contamination will not keep antibody levels high. Blood tests may fluctuate up and down for several reasons, including the use of different laboratories. But, these fluctuations should not be dramatic if gluten is not being ingested.

Nevertheless, serological tests are not sensitive markers of bowel recovery or dietary indiscretion. In fact, they are very gross markers of the latter. The only true measure of compliance and improvement is the diagnostic standard, the intestinal biopsy.

Follow-Up Biopsy

Many experts feel that a follow-up biopsy should be done to document healing. It is not now necessary to establish the diagnosis, but many experts want to document that the villous atrophy and inflammatory changes have improved. We have shown that the presence of persistent villous atrophy is associated with an increased risk of malignancies and fractures. Typically, biopsy results take longer to normalize than blood tests, but some people have biopsies that normalize rapidly and completely. They also tend to normalize from the distal (lower) part of the small intestine up. Biopsies taken from the proximal (upper) section of the intestine—where they are routinely taken—will, therefore, be the last to change.

This may not apply to small children. Because antibody testing is less reliable in infants and young children, a follow-up biopsy may be recommended to confirm the diagnosis, document improvement on the diet, and monitor progress. But follow-up biopsies on children are not typically performed.

Since the longer you are on the diet, the greater the improvement, a follow-up biopsy after two to five years on the diet should be sufficient. If this biopsy shows no improvement, it is most likely due to ongoing gluten ingestion or another condition.

If blood tests are negative but the biopsy remains positive, it may be because a different pathologist is reading the results. Patients should request that an expert GI pathologist compare their follow-up biopsy with their original biopsy. This may involve some inconvenience on the part of the physician, but it is important for the patient.

Other reasons for conducting a follow-up biopsy include:

- Patients work very hard at the diet. They often wish to see how they are doing, and blood tests are not a reliable indicator of intestinal improvement.
- People with no symptoms are hard to evaluate. For them, the follow-up biopsy may be particularly appropriate. Many experts recommend it in these cases, but there are no studies showing its value.
- People who have persistent or recurrent symptoms while on the diet may have negative antibodies. It is hard to determine what is going on without a biopsy. Many of these patients are worried they may have a lymphoma or an enteropathy associated with a lymphoma. Biopsy can rule this out.

Patients with persistent symptoms will have more biopsies and these should be compared with previous biopsies to indicate whether people are truly on the diet and the exact nature of the improvement. These patients also need to exclude other conditions such as collagenous sprue, lymphoma, bacterial overgrowth, or pancreatic insufficiency. A colonoscopy is necessary to rule out lymphocytic colitis.

Patients who change physicians or see a specialist for an opinion should bring old biopsy results or have them forwarded. It is very important for new physicians to review the biopsy with a pathologist familiar with celiac disease. Reading the biopsy report is not sufficient.

Repeating the biopsy is of no value unless:

1. The previous biopsy is reviewed for celiac disease; it may just require another pathologist to identify it.
2. The original biopsy is available for comparison with newer biopsies.

If these steps were followed more often, the added expense and inconvenience of a repeat biopsy and endoscopy might be avoided. Biopsy slides are retained by pathologists for years, by law.

Family Testing

It must be on your father's side. (Anonymous)

Everyone in my family has presented so differently. My mother had neuropathies. She was having an endoscopy for reflux and they discovered the celiac disease. My sister had anemia that she couldn't get controlled and started to lose a great deal of weight. She is biopsy proven (to have celiac disease). My daughter was silent—she was diagnosed at thirteen with celiac disease as part of a family screening—she had no symptoms and a totally flat biopsy. But she had osteopenia on a bone scan. None of us were the same. (Laura, 43)

Children and first-degree relatives of patients positively diagnosed with celiac disease should have blood tests for the condition whether or not they have symptoms. Nevertheless, there are many emotional as well as physical issues involved in family testing that often delay or derail the process.

Celiac disease runs in families and should be diagnosed early before complications can arise. Initially, this involves only blood testing (recommended for children after the age of five to seven) that is repeated every five years, or in the presence of symptoms.

Studies have shown that the prevalence of celiac disease is up to 10 percent in first-degree relatives. A recent study of siblings with celiac disease was even more vivid. In families where at least two siblings have been diagnosed with celiac disease, the prevalence of celiac disease in other siblings was double that estimate. Offspring and more distant relatives were also at higher risk (15 percent of offspring, 20 percent of second-degree relatives, and 17 percent of first cousins). This result was attributed to the potential for a common gene in each family.

High-Risk Group Testing

There is good evidence that children with type 1 diabetes (IDDM), children with Down syndrome, and first-degree relatives who initially have negative blood work may become positive some years later. We recommend that these at-risk groups have repeat testing every three to five years if the initial serology is negative.

Genetic Testing

My son is negative at twelve years old; when should I test again?
(Ron, 37)

Genetic testing can help to determine which family members are extremely unlikely to develop the disease. If family members do have the genes, they should be tested again if they develop symptoms or at an appropriate interval, usually every five years.

There are specific genes that have been identified in celiac disease. These genes are responsible for the HLA-DQ2 and HLA-DQ8 molecules that are required to express the disease. (See A Genetic Primer—Fitting the Groove, Chapter 6.) It is believed that other genes, not yet identified, are important. Testing for HLA-DQ2 and HLA-DQ8 is highly sensitive but poorly specific, since approximately 30 percent of the general population have these genes. Having them does not necessarily indicate that someone will develop celiac disease. But, if someone does *not* have these genes, it is virtually impossible that they do or will have celiac disease.

Genetic testing can be extremely useful to:

1. Eliminate family members who initially have negative blood work from repeated testing for celiac disease
2. Test patients who are already on a gluten-free diet who do not want to be subjected to a gluten challenge

Genetic testing is not used to diagnose celiac disease, but it is a useful test in certain situations that can *eliminate* celiac disease from the clinical spectrum.

Genetic Home Test Kits

Genetic testing that includes testing for celiac disease genes is now available through home testing companies. These tests require the user to spit into a container, which is then sent to a lab for analysis. Unlike the existing blood and cheek swab tests where results are sent to the physician, the results of these tests are returned directly to the consumer.

Used commonly to determine ancestry, some companies give genetic results for medical conditions.

Because the home genetic test bypasses the physician, it raises a number of controversial issues:

1. The test may be overused, causing unnecessary concern, since few genetically predisposed individuals actually develop celiac disease.
2. There may be a lack of support from the patients' physicians for assistance in interpretation of the results.
3. There is no insurance coverage for home gene tests.
4. There is a lack of knowledge among many physicians of the HLA significance in celiac disease.

As with any type of home test, the importance of the results depends on how the patient uses the information. The presence of the HLA gene does *not* indicate the condition, only an at-risk state. (For more on testing devices for gluten, see Glutenostics–Gluten Detective Rapid Urine/Stool Test, Chapter 4, and The Nima Device, Chapter 21.)

Video Capsule Endoscopy

Video capsule endoscopy has an emerging role in the evaluation and follow-up of people diagnosed with celiac disease. Currently, the only approved indications are for chronic gastrointestinal bleeding and Crohn's disease.

In this test, the patient swallows a pill-sized camera that projects video images onto a small monitor that is fitted to a harness on the body. The camera, which is the size of a large vitamin pill, is triggered before being ingested. Children are capable of taking the "pill" and have been trained to swallow a jelly bean whole in preparation for the procedure. The camera is capable of taking almost fifty thousand images and travels most of the small intestine for about eight hours.

Capsule endoscopy is being evaluated in the diagnosis of celiac disease, especially in people with complicated celiac disease (including those with abdominal pain and bleeding), as well as the elderly, or people diagnosed in childhood who have been on a regular diet. It is felt that this latter group is at an increased risk of developing cancer. It can show the extent of celiac disease, how far down the intestine it has progressed, and whether there are polyps, ulcers, or cancers. Ulceration might account for pain or blood in the stool, and suspicious lesions can be biopsied in a separate procedure.

Capsule endoscopy offers people with complications a relatively noninvasive follow-up for medical assessment. The exact role of capsule endoscopy has to be determined. It is, however, an exciting procedure with great potential for the management of patients with celiac disease.

PART IV

THE DIET: DO YOU EAT TO LIVE OR LIVE TO EAT?

Each is given a bag of tools,
A shapeless mass and a book of rules;
And each must make, ere life is flown,
A stumbling block or a stepping-stone.

—R. L. Sharpe

Getting diagnosed is the first big hurdle. Mastering the gluten-free diet is the next hurdle, and it is a tall one. When you leave the doctor's office and start to navigate the real world of gluten-free living, there are many skills to learn and details to master. You will require a "toolbox" that should include:

1. An understanding of which grains, ingredients, and foods are safe and which are not
2. The ability to read labels
3. A knowledge of the areas in the gluten-free diet that are unclear and the science that is available that will enable you to make educated, personal choices
4. The ability to question waiters, caterers, hostesses, or school lunchroom cooks and advocate for yourself in order to obtain a safe and satisfying meal
5. Patience—with family, friends, and strangers who may (or may not) cope as well as you will with the gluten-free diet
6. A focus on *healthy,* not just gluten-free, eating
7. Adherence to the diet that enhances, not interferes with, quality of life

These tools are the stepping-stones to enable you to enjoy, rather than suffer through, a gluten-free life.

18

What Living Gluten-Free Really Means: The Basics

Practice yourself in little things; . . . and thence proceed to greater.

—*Epictetus*

I was standing there with my orange juice and bagel and the doctor said: "I've got good news and bad news. That's your last bagel, but I know what's wrong with you." (Heather, 43)

"You must never eat gluten again." It sounds simple enough—until you realize that gluten is hidden in, around, and all over the supermarket and drugstore. Pizza, pasta, bread, and beer are the obvious, but not the only, suspects.

Many patients want definitive answers: "Can I eat this, or not?" But, the safety of some foods is still unclear. And, more important, eating and living gluten-free does not simply consist of memorizing a list of "forbidden" and "safe" foods—or sticking to fifteen to twenty "safe" products until you can no longer stand eating them. There is no need to eliminate the wide variety of fresh, healthy food that is still available to you.

Although the gluten-free diet is not that easy to master, it is less difficult than it may first appear. Do not expect to be an expert or excel overnight, or within the first month. It takes time and practice. Everyone has an "oops" or two (or more). Without doubt, a sense of humor speeds the learning and living process.

How Much Is Too Much?

Eating gluten is like falling down and scraping your knee. You damage the knee, but in time it heals. If you keep falling down and reinjuring your knee every day, it's never going to heal. Similarly, the more gluten you eat, the greater the inflammation and possible damage.

We know that ingesting an eighth of a teaspoon of flour causes visible intestinal damage. We do not know what happens to the intestine with smaller amounts such as the chronic ingestion of bread crumbs in a butter dish.

We do not know how much gluten you must eat—or how often—for that damage to accumulate. We don't know if that crumb in the dish is a scrape, a bruise, or continual damage. So you must be diligent on the issues of cross contamination and "cheating." (Anne Lee, R.D.)

Living gluten-free (GF) means eliminating all foods containing even a trace amount of the grains containing gluten. That includes foods made with derivatives of those grains or additives and stabilizers containing those grains.

Grain Science

The grain families and their genetic makeup have been researched and described in great depth. Grains are divided into various classes, subclasses, orders, families, and species. Each branch of the grain "tree" contains a slightly different genetic makeup and protein sequence that determines its properties and, for people with celiac disease, its toxicity. (See Figure 7, page 22.)

Celiac disease is triggered by certain grains, specifically those that contain gluten, a term that is generally used to include all of the toxic protein portions found in wheat (gliadins), rye (secalins), and barley (hordeins). Specifically, that includes those in the following box:

GRAINS TO AVOID

Wheat (wheat germ, wheat bran)

Rye

Barley (barley malt)

Faro

Bulgur

Couscous

Spelt

Kamut

Semolina

Triticale

Einkorn

Some grasses belong to different branches of the plant tree and are not toxic to people with celiac disease.

GRAINS THAT ARE SAFE

Rice

Corn

Millet

Teff

Sorghum

Wild rice

Buckwheat (despite the name)

Quinoa

Amaranth

See Appendix B for a more complete explanation of grains.

Wheat Starch

Wheat starch consists of wheat that has had the gluten portion "washed out." When wheat starch is used in a food labeled "gluten-free," it must appear in the ingredients list and meet the Food and Drug Administration (FDA) requirements of less than 20 ppm (parts per million)* for gluten-free foods. When the ingredients list says only "starch," it means cornstarch.

A special grade of wheat starch is permitted on the gluten-free diet—and is used on food labels marked "gluten-free." The international standards for gluten-free foods were revised in 2014.† They contain two categories of "Foods for Special Dietary Use for Persons Intolerant to Gluten." The first category includes foods labeled "gluten-free" and consists of foods with a gluten level that "does not exceed 20mg/kg in total."

The second category includes foods that are "specially processed to reduce gluten content to a level above 20 up to 100mg/kg." Wheat starch is an example of this type of ingredient. The label to be used on this second category of foods will be determined by each European country and may include designations such as "very low gluten." Any foods sold in the United States must meet the FDA requirements for "gluten-free" food labels. (For more, see Chapter 19.)

Are Trace Amounts Acceptable?

There is an ongoing scientific discussion regarding the safe threshold for "residual" gluten in products labeled and/or considered gluten-free. As we have noted, it is still not clear what effect small amounts of gluten have on the long-term health of a patient with celiac disease. Some naturally occurring gluten-free foods do, in fact, contain trace amounts of gluten.

The gluten-free diet in Finland is considered to have up to 30 milligrams of gluten per day (a slice of regular bread has 2.25 grams). In a recent Finnish study, all celiacs on this diet improved and showed a normal longevity without an increased risk of cancer. Therefore, re-

---

* Parts per million is the current standard for evaluating amounts of gluten in food and correlates with extremely small amounts. Twenty ppm is 20/1,000,000 or .002 percent

† Commission Implementing Regulation (EC) No. 41/2009 [EU] No. 828/2014

searchers believe that these trace amounts are tolerated well by *most* people with celiac disease.

Some researchers have conducted a gluten challenge (see Gluten Challenge, Chapter 4) with patients in order to ascertain how much gluten must be ingested before the intestinal mucosa shows inflammation and damage. Results have been inconclusive because:

- The studies have been mainly short-term and the results have not been uniform.
- Most people tolerate 10 milligrams of gluten, but not 100 milligrams.
- Some individuals are more sensitive than others to even minute amounts of gluten. The amount of intestinal damage is extremely varied in people with celiac disease, even on diagnosis, and recovery also varies.
- It is unclear what level of inflammatory response is harmful on a long-term basis.

Rigorous scientific studies have not been conducted that examine a large enough population over a long enough period of time and take into account the potential for noncompliance and/or cross contamination.

In clinical practice, a lack of symptoms does not necessarily mean a lack of inflammation.

Until the data is more conclusive, we recommend that people attempt to ingest "no detectable amounts" of gluten—insofar as that is achievable.

Oats

Oats remain a dilemma for some patients despite the fact that a good deal of scientific research has focused on this food source. While the grain was formerly considered unsafe for people with celiac disease, it is now considered safe for most.

The protein in oats—the part containing the *avenin** protein fraction—was shown to cause a reaction in a few celiac patients that is

---

* The offending protein fractions in wheat are *gliadins,* in rye *secalins,* and in barley *hordeins.*

not fundamentally different from the reaction to gluten peptides. But clinical studies have shown that the majority of people with celiac disease tolerate oats quite well. Therefore, it is believed that oats—as a grain—are safe for most individuals with celiac disease, but may cause a reaction in some. Studies have found that patients ingesting oats sometimes have more symptoms due to the increase of dietary fiber, but very few have any type of immune reaction.

We advise using oats because (1) the scientific evidence supports this approach, and (2) oats add both fiber and variety to the gluten-free diet—elements that are frequently lacking.

Cross contamination is an issue. Oats and other grains are often grown, stored, and/or processed on common land and facilities. Recent studies have shown that some cross contamination can occur. But it is unclear whether the amount of cross contamination of oats by wheat is sufficient to cause harm to people with celiac disease. The amount of gluten found in certain brands of commercial oats is extremely small. But it is also important to take into account the amount of contamination from other foods that someone may be getting on a daily basis. Some patients with celiac disease and dermatitis herpetiformis cannot tolerate even minute amounts of gluten.

It is important that any oats eaten by those with celiac disease be declared gluten-free by the manufacturer, one that mills and packages oats on dedicated machinery. And patients who consume oats on a consistent basis should be monitored with annual blood tests and have appropriately timed follow-up biopsies.

Cross Contamination

They have these elaborate breakfasts (in Sweden). I always bring my gluten-free cereal, so all I need is milk. But they had a table with all breads and on the top shelf they had a little basket and it said "gluten-free." I didn't eat it just because I'm so neurotic. . . . I didn't know how they cut it and if it was contaminated. (Dan, 53)

Cross contamination is an important issue whether you are in your own kitchen or out and about. For people with dermatitis herpetiformis who may be exquisitely sensitive to gluten, cross contamination can be an especially difficult problem.

Grains other than oats are also subject to contamination. Some cornmeal and rice flour is mixed with other grains in different manufactured products. (This should be on the label.) Corn and rice are safe; mixtures may not be. Other grains such as buckwheat may be processed in or near equipment used for grains containing gluten. People are urged to buy grains from mills that are either dedicated to gluten-free products or recommended by knowledgeable sources.

There are a few guidelines that may help in avoiding potential cross contamination. They are easier to implement and follow at home than when eating in the real world.

Basic Rules for Avoiding Cross Contamination

Soap and Water Rule

Water has been around for millions of years, soap for many hundreds. They were paired for good reason and can keep cutting boards, cooking utensils, and hands free of gluten. Use them liberally, and teach children to use them—they may be the cheapest part of the gluten-free diet. New studies show that pots and pans washed with soap and water can be made safe for use.

Separate or Duplicate

Set aside separate cutting boards for gluten ingredients if they are used regularly in your house so that kids and visitors know where to work with unsafe crumbs. Mesh colanders and individual-compartment toasters are hard to clean. If you make pasta dishes and toast regularly, either use nonmesh stainless steel colanders and toaster ovens with racks that wash well, or keep "gluten" and "gluten-free" versions. Rule 1 applies to everything else.

Don't Double-Dip and Mix Serving Utensils

If a serving utensil goes in a jar/can/dish, touches "gluten food," and goes back in the jar/can/dish, it is off-limits. Tell the family: "If you double-dip it, you own it; I get my own peanut butter/jelly/butter/salsa." At someone's house or in a restaurant, assume these items are contaminated unless you see them opened.

If you are out at a salad bar or buffet, serving spoon swapping is common. See what is bordering the dish and make an informed decision as to what you should eat.

Stay On It

Be aware that contamination is often "on," not "in," the food.

Frying Oil. One of the biggest pitfalls in a restaurant is the oil pot. Chefs routinely keep oil at a boil for all of their fried foods. Baskets containing the items to be flash fried are then dipped, cooked, and drained. Breading and coating from fried items such as calamari, Buffalo wings, and mozzarella sticks remain in the oil to contaminate the french fries as they make their trip through the pot. Ask if the fries are cooked in the same oil as other breaded items and avoid fried items if you are unsure.

Look for Dust. Flour keeps ingredients from sticking together. It may be used to "dust" dried fruit and coat baking pans. Pastry chefs and waiters may forget that the "flourless" chocolate cake is made in a pan dusted with butter and flour when they recite the ingredients to you. Be observant, even in your own home and in the homes of friends. And don't be afraid to ask questions.

Get Expert Advice. Talk to nutritionists/dieticians, support group counselors, and the parents of children with celiac disease about cross contamination. They have learned to navigate school lunchrooms, restaurants, parties, and dozens of other social situations where cross contamination may be an issue. Learn from their experience.

> My girlfriend had her ten-year-old tested for celiac disease. I told her, "What took me two and a half years to learn, I can set up for you in a week." (Sue, 41)

Don't Crawl Under a Rock. Food will be contaminated. As explained above, it has not been scientifically determined whether the minuscule amounts of gluten that a diligent person inadvertently ingests have a negative, long-term effect on their health. All that one can do is be careful and cautious, learn what and how to eat safely, then get up and out. **It is important that you not let the gluten-free diet run or ruin your life. There needs to be a balance.**

Are You Getting Good Information?

A great deal of the information compiled about the gluten-free diet began within the celiac community. Some of it is excellent; some of it truly inaccurate. There are also myths about foods to avoid that refuse to die and must be dispelled if patients are to enjoy the large amount of safe, commercial products. **Be aware: there are some people who claim to be on a "strict" gluten-free diet that is not really gluten-free. Yet they are strictly adherent to it! This is a greater problem than cross contamination.**

In a recent study websites with information about celiac disease and gluten-free food were shown to contain a disturbing amount of misinformation. Of the sites evaluated (forty-one were in the United States, ten in Britain, two in Canada, seven in Australia/New Zealand, one in Ireland), almost 16 percent had inaccuracies. While the preponderance of the sites had accurate information, too many did not, and many were incomplete. Focusing on scientific information where the sources are transparent (well documented from doctors, nutritionists, experts, and professionals listed and/or on staff) and the information is regularly updated is crucial. There must be more than "we feel that this is unsafe" or "we regard a food as containing gluten until proved otherwise." Being conservative about the diet is not necessarily good advice if there is no scientific rationale for the restrictions.

Health Food Stores

I was told, in no uncertain terms, that the spelt cake that was on special was gluten-free. That spelt was a gluten-free grain and totally safe for someone with celiac disease. He really seemed to know what he was talking about—at least he believed what he was telling me. (Sharon, 54)

The information and products available at health food stores are often far from healthy for someone with celiac disease. The cross contamination of foods stored in open bins, supplements that are incorrectly labeled, and information on what is gluten-free may all be risky. Make sure that you get your information from a medically reliable source, not a health food store employee. (And spelt is wheat no matter how it is spell't.)

SUMMING UP THE BASICS

1. Aim for "no detectable amounts of gluten" in everything you make or eat.

2. Expand your knowledge of grains.

3. Learn about cross contamination. This is a tool that requires the most vigilance. Look for it in and on the foods you stock at home and those you eat when out.

4. Understand that it is very difficult, if not impossible, to avoid all gluten at all times. Be diligent, but realistic.

19

Reading Labels

I had never heard of gluten before—hydrolyzed protein, dextrin, di-
glycerides, citric acid: these were very foreign things to me. I'm not
a chemist, I'm just a mother. (Sue, 41)

Forty years ago, Betty Furness changed the food landscape. She suc-
ceeded in getting manufacturers to label the salt and sugar they liberally
added to their jars of baby food to appeal to mom's taste testing. Consumer awareness entered a new age.

People with celiac disease are very special consumers. Along with
people with virulent food allergies, they must rely on food labels to stay
healthy. Unfortunately, until recently, navigating these tiny pieces of
paper required more than a magnifying glass. Patients also needed a
knowledge of chemistry and food science.

The 2014 Labeling Law

Today, labeling laws are again being changed in an exciting way.
Wheat is taking its place alongside other known food allergens as a
targeted "poison" for some consumers. The Food Allergen Labeling and
Consumer Protection Act was signed into law in 2004, and amended
to describe labeling guidelines for gluten-free foods in 2013. It requires all food labels to state whether a product contains one of the
eight major foods or food groups that account for the majority of
food allergies, including:

Milk	Fish
Eggs	Crustacean shellfish

| Tree nuts | Wheat |
| Peanuts | Soybeans |

This will make it far easier for patients with celiac disease to read a label and identify potential problems in the alphabet soup of additives and ingredients. Although the current law does not go far enough for people with celiac disease, who still require a knowledge of other potential sources of gluten (e.g., barley, commonly seen as "malt"), it is a huge step forward.

Labels 101

The materials are indifferent, but the use we make of them is not a matter of indifference.

—Epictetus

It is imperative that patients with celiac disease be well versed in the specific ingredients that may contain gluten, or its derivatives, in order to make informed buying decisions. We need to know when a label is "safe," when it is questionable and requires a call to the manufacturer, and when to leave the product on the market shelf.

It is equally important to have this knowledge when food is marinated or basted with a sauce and the food preparer, caterer, or chef offers the bottle or can for inspection. You should be able to determine, on the spot, if the dish is "safe" to eat.

The ingredients on a label are listed in descending order of volume in the product, and by the time you reach line three or four, you are examining extremely small amounts. If the label is longer than that, you are probably ingesting more test tube products than real food.

For people with celiac disease, the key to reading labels is finding any hidden gluten. The list of suspicious ingredients, once you have eliminated the obvious suspects, is surprisingly short.

Ingredients and Additives Worth Understanding

There has been a great deal of controversy about ingredients in the celiac disease community. A list and explanation of safe and forbidden ingredients can be found in Appendix A. It includes:

Caramel color

Citric acid

Dextrin

Dextrose

Flavors (artificial and natural)

Glucose syrup

Guar gum

Herbs

Hydrolyzed plant protein
    (HPP)

Hydrolyzed vegetable protein
    (HVP)

Malt

Maltodextrin

Modified food starch

Mono- and diglycerides

MSG

Oat gum

Seasonings

Seitan

Soy sauce

Spices

Starch

Vanilla

Vinegar

Whey

Yeast

Some of these ingredients will be clearly listed under the 2014 law as to their wheat content. Also, studies have proved that some of the listed ingredients have always been safe (e.g., distilled vinegar) but their "forbidden" reputation lives on!

With an understanding of ingredients, you can then approach cooking in your own kitchen, shopping, and eating in the real world with greater confidence.

Gluten-Free Labels

The FDA, which regulates and watches over these matters, has adopted a standard that permits no more than 20 parts per million in a product that is labeled "gluten-free." The European standard designated by the Codex Alimentarius allows no more than 20 ppm on products labeled "gluten-free." Any food labeled "gluten-free" coming into the United States will have to meet U.S. standards.

Made in a Facility That Processes Wheat Products

There is currently one advisory label that can present a confusing warning:

"May be processed in a facility that processes wheat products or on shared equipment"

Some patients who are very sensitive to even small amounts of gluten may be more hesitant to eat products made on shared equipment. However, any food labeled "gluten-free," whether or not it also contains an advisory statement, must meet all the requirements of the FDA final rule. If the product is something you eat regularly, you should contact the manufacturer or consult with your health care providers.

Several things are important to understand. First, not all products will say "gluten-free." Many, in fact, will be gluten-free without that designation. Second, because of testing and cross-contamination issues, it is sometimes difficult to ensure that a product marked "gluten-free" actually is.

Testing for Gluten in a Product

It is difficult, if not impossible, to scientifically ascertain if a product is completely gluten-free, especially in grains that may have cross contamination because of manufacturing practices. This is because:

1. Manufacturers do not test every box or bag of a given food on an assembly line.
2. Amounts can—and do—vary within any given product line, i.e., in different packages of oats.
3. Current tests are reliable down to approximately 20 parts per million. Therefore, food scientists currently designate a food to have "no discernible amount" of gluten below that level.

Complicating the matter further is the issue of test kits. Similar to the issues with blood (serology) testing, there are varying specificities and controls between the kits. As of this writing, the FDA has not endorsed one method of testing. The celiac disease patient (the consumer in this case) is therefore left to decide how to interpret the results. The FDA recommends that "consumers with celiac disease and others sensitive to gluten consult with their health care providers for advice about whether the criteria followed by any specific gluten-free certification program would meet their individual needs."

The Bottom Line

1. Different patients may have differing degrees of sensitivity and/or tolerance to small amounts of gluten ingestion.
2. The concept of ppm in any given product does not take into account (a) the amount/portion of the product eaten every day or every week, (b) the other products with similar amounts of gluten eaten by that person that day, or (c) the cross contamination that person is exposed to.

Therefore, we recommend that to remain healthy, people learn how to read labels in order to find hidden gluten and aim for "none."

Labels–The Next Steps

Reassess Your Kitchen Pantry

If you, or a member of the family, are newly diagnosed, start your label reading at home. Whether the family decision is to go completely gluten-free or simply to separate foods, it is important to review the labels on every can and jar. Isolate cans and jars with gluten and/or questionable ingredients. Some people may choose to eliminate jars with obvious gluten. Consider donating those food items to an appropriate charitable organization.

There is no need to throw out every can and jar you own and start all over. Reassess does not necessarily mean eliminate.

Research the Products You or Your Children Eat Regularly

If you are going to eat something regularly, make sure it is safe. If you love a certain product and are unsure of its status, call the manufacturer. There are resources on the web, professionals, and support groups that can help in this process. **Ultimately, it is up to you to take charge of your own eating and feel comfortable making calls directly.** As wheat derivatives and gluten become more well known to the food manufacturers, this process should become easier.

You must be more wary of highly processed foods. The labels of low-fat, no-fat, and "diet" foods often include a list of chemicals as long as the jar. The chemicals are necessary to make these foods palatable without the salt, fat, and sugar that normally do the job.

Check Ingredients Regularly

Ingredients change. Do not stop checking labels, even on foods you have been buying regularly. Get in the habit of reading labels and keeping up to date on celiac disease literature and food items.

Everything Does Not Have to Say "Gluten-Free"

Many brand-name products are safe to eat. That is, you do not have to buy "gluten-free" everything. Many commercial salad dressings, mustards, tomato sauces, ketchups, candy bars, etc., are safe as is.

Patients with Diabetes and Celiac Disease Need to Read Labels for "Carbs"

Patients who have diabetes also have to read labels to understand the change in carbohydrate levels in gluten-free food. The standard for carb counting is: one carb equals 15 grams. So one slice of wheat bread is usually one carb. Unfortunately, this does not translate for the gluten-free diet. One slice of gluten-free bread is usually more than one carb. Patients must learn that the amount of insulin must come up or the serving size must come down.

You Need Consistency

Products need to be consistent to be safe. If you get a product from company X and you get sick from it, call them. If you do not get a clear answer, or one that is different from your previous contact with the company, that becomes an inconsistent and unacceptable product.

Learn to Tell the Forest from the Trees

There are patients who spend a great deal of time focusing on the chemical names of ingredients on a label—and then eat products (e.g., rice cereals) made with barley malt. While focusing on trace amounts (the tiny trees), they are missing the forest—and often have intestinal biopsies that do not return to normal.

Questions That Remain

Blue or Veined Cheeses

Stilton cheese is traditionally made (i.e., "veined") with a starter consisting of bread mold. Similarly, to start the fermentation of "real"

Roquefort, a mixture of bread crumbs is sprinkled over the surface of the starter cheese. It is unclear whether or not the bread is broken down by the mold and whether toxic peptides (of gliadin) remain. Thus, in the absence of scientific data, Roquefort and Stilton are questionable cheeses.

If you are buying commercially made blue cheese (gorgonzola, blue) in the United States, it may be made with a chemical starter, which is generally safe. Read the label.

If you are eating out or traveling abroad, approach the cheese tray, as well as salads and dishes made or sprinkled with blue cheeses, with some care. Other cheeses that may contain gluten include beer cheese and ale cheese.

Highly processed cheeses (nonblue) and low-fat cheeses may also contain gluten. As in most food areas, fresh is best.

Low-Fat, No-Fat, Low-Carb, No-Carb Mania

People who have been eating highly processed low-fat, no-carb foods may encounter label shock when first diagnosed with celiac disease. Food scientists are continually creating new "tastes" in the test tube to fool our taste buds into believing we're eating the real thing. Stabilizers—some gluten-based—are needed to keep the chemicals that compose the product together in the jar and in your mouth.

If it says "low" or "non" fat/carb, read the label *very* carefully.

Reading labels can be fun. Armed with good information, you do not have to be a chemist to understand them.

Looking for Glues

Very few people grow the food they eat. Produced all around the world, our food supply is raised, farmed, harvested, treated, packaged, and shipped to our local stores. We do not always know what is in or on our food in addition to the raw material. An example of this is the use of an enzyme in processed foods that has been shown to be more toxic to people with celiac disease.

The production of certain processed foods requires emulsifiers and substances that can cross-link food proteins, or hold the food together. One such product is the enzyme microbial transglutaminase (eTG), a cousin to the tissue transglutaminase that is the autoantigen—the culprit—in celiac disease. (See What Is Tissue Transglutaminase [tTG]?,

Chapter 2.) It has many applications in processed food production. It is marketed to bind meat and fish pieces; to keep the liquid from separating out of yogurt, ice cream, and cheese with a low fat content; and to keep the soft texture of tofu. It is part of an arsenal of additives that enable food manufacturers to increase the texture, shelf life, and appearance of their products.

While it is unknown how widely this enzyme is used, a recent study done in the Netherlands showed that eating food treated with eTG can enhance the immune response of people with celiac disease.

This is an area that requires more research if we are to fully understand the causes of celiac disease, why it is becoming more common, and what we should—and should not—be eating to treat the condition.

HELPFUL HINTS

1. Locate retail stores and Internet and mail-order resources where you can buy gluten-free food that you can trust.

2. Shop more often for fresh food.

3. Taste lots of gluten-free products and develop a shopping list of the ones that you enjoy.

4. Keep updated on new developments and gluten-free products.

5. Enjoy what you do eat.

20

Cooking Without Gluten

When my two-year-old daughter was first diagnosed, we only fed her boiled chicken, milk, and rice. I was scared to death to give her anything to eat. (Sue, 41)

Some people cook Italian, some people cook Irish, some people cook Armenian, and some people cook gluten-free. It's just another way of designing your kitchen. (George Chookosian, Foods by George)

The comedienne Totie Fields had a signature comedy routine that explained why she was a terrible cook. When first married, she said, she told her husband that she wanted to please him in every way, but could excel in only *one* room of the house. He could have his pick. She would pause and deadpan—"He didn't pick the kitchen."

The kitchen takes on new meaning when someone in the house has celiac disease. Whether you consider cooking an art, a chore, or someone else's responsibility, the safest place to eat is usually at home, where preparation and cross contamination can be controlled.

Cooking Styles

Cooking starts with your "kitchen style." While many people will do several of the following at any given time, most fall into one of these categories out of necessity or choice.

Do you usually:

- Cook for yourself and your family
- Reheat frozen or packaged meals

- Order in
- Eat out

Whatever your style prior to diagnosis, cooking—or at the very least "assembling"—should become an important part of the learning curve. And as you reassess what goes into your mouth—from the stove, the oven, the local takeout, the supermarket freezer, or a restaurant— you must think about nutrition as well as "gluten-free." **It is crucial for people on a lifelong gluten-free diet to focus on the "healthy" part of cooking and eating.**

The Cook

I've started baking and had some messes and some successes. More successes than messes, really. The head of our support group gave me a recipe for apple pie that is delicious. I make it all the time. (Heather, 43)

My wife knows more about what I should and shouldn't eat than I do. (Fred, 63)

If you or a family member cooks regularly, you will be eating a wider variety of food more rapidly. Unless you are baking, which involves a real change in ingredients and amounts, mastering gluten-free cooking is mainly substitution and common sense.

If you have a large book of recipes and favorite dishes, you will find it surprisingly easy to adapt them. A wide variety of gluten-free flours, pastas, breads and baked goods, soy sauces, and soup stocks are available. All natural spices are gluten-free.

Lasagna, moussaka, spaghetti and meatballs, casseroles, stews, soups, and cookies can all be made gluten-free—and frozen—without any more effort than making the old variety. When you adapt, and substitute, think about lowering the fat and increasing the fiber content.

The Reheater

I come home exhausted, my feet are killing me—do I want to start cooking? No way. (Linda, 62)

If most meals in your house consist of warming up frozen or packaged foods, you may find fewer already prepared gluten-free meals on the market. Gluten-free alternatives are available—and every year there are more manufacturers entering the market—but your choices are more limited. Also, frozen meals may have a high level of fat and fewer nutrients/fiber than the home-cooked variety. You might want to start cooking and freezing your own gluten-free creations.

Taking Out and Ordering In

If you pick up fast food on the way home, or regularly use takeout, you may have to rethink your meal planning. Fast food and takeout are not necessarily safe, or healthy. While work and school schedules may dictate the choices for those whose kitchen depends on the cooking ability of others, think about making and stocking your kitchen with home-made gluten-free choices that can be reheated at the last minute. You will be expanding your eating choices as well as eating healthier meals.

Eating Out

If all that you ever make for dinner is reservations, see Restaurants, Chapter 21. Increasingly, there are restaurants that cater to those who eat gluten-free, but that grouping is still small.

People who eat out regularly will spend the time and energy to cultivate safe and enjoyable eating experiences. But eating gluten-free is not as safe or easy in the real world, and you will find your own kitchen increasingly important.

For the time that you do spend in the kitchen, some of the suggestions below may be helpful.

Cooking Gluten-Free

No matter what your kitchen style, it is important that people with celiac disease learn to cook and eat well-balanced meals. Not just to regain what they lost after months or years of malabsorption, but to stay healthy.

Learning to cook gluten-free is a process: it does not come with a fast-forward button. But, it does not have to mean starting over from scratch. While there are many excellent cookbooks, baking books, and website recipes dedicated to "gluten-free," your old cookbooks can be easily adapted. The approach should be similar to that with canned goods: you do not have to toss everything and start all over. Ethnic cookbooks have many naturally gluten-free recipes.

THINGS TO REMEMBER

Do not isolate the family—or the patient—by completely changing what they are eating. *Modify and adapt* what they are used to.

If you have a split kitchen in which some family members are eating gluten-free and others are not, plan meals ahead so that there is as much overlap as possible.

Be adventurous.

- Try different gluten-free grains.

- Keep tasting different gluten-free products—new ones regularly come on the market. Vendors attend support groups and celiac disease events with free samples.

- Experiment with ethnic dishes, which are often fast and easy to make.

- Try cooking. You might enjoy it.

- Allow young children with celiac disease to cook, control, and enjoy a gluten-free kitchen.

- Plan ahead and stock your refrigerator, cabinets, and freezer with gluten-free products and meals so you are not eating a can of tuna or gluten-free cereal every night. There are now a wide variety of different gluten-free foods (breads, cakes, crackers, snacks) that cater to many different tastes and preferences.

- Stock your car, backpack, or desk with gluten-free snacks so they are always "at hand."

- Think choice, not restriction.

Ceil, my wife, was diagnosed in 1990 and there was little to eat. I always wanted to learn more about baking. So I went to the library and looked up what the allowable ingredients were and what they brought to the party. I researched gluten and what it did to the final structure of whatever it was in. Then I came up with a few different mixes. Every day I researched gluten-free ingredients and made all the formulas I use today from that.

I had pages and pages and pages of drawings. I would draw an arc (the dome of the bread), and I would measure how high the bread rose with each formula, bake time, oven temperature, etc. I would see which one rose the highest and tasted the best. Ceil's family were good taste testers—we threw a lot out. The birds and squirrels took it away.

Today, people are looking for a consistent product—whether in a mix, a box, or a bag. People don't have the time to do that kind of experimenting. And it's expensive. Most people want the mixes and finished product.

After doing all the groundwork, teaching myself the chemistry of the components, learning mixes, and getting them on the market, I got a degree at the Culinary Institute of America. They had no experience with gluten-free food—no class, no recipes, no formulas. They felt: "Who wants to eat like that anyway?" I spent nine months at the CIA learning the craft of baking, the techniques. Then I developed the baked line of products.

Now, my mentor for traditional bread baking is teaching gluten-free baking classes. And I'm invited as a guest lecturer and commencement speaker.

Our thoughts on navigating your own gluten-free kitchen?

1. Don't be afraid to fail. Try things more than once. Chemical research is not necessary, but you have to put a lot of effort into it.
2. Food is the treatment—that's the positive news. There are so many products a person with celiac disease can eat.
3. Try not to go nuts in your kitchen; be logical. You don't need two sets of everything—that's why you have soap and water. The head person in the kitchen has to do what's easiest for him or her in terms of a gluten-free kitchen.

4. *Use your imagination. People come in and say they miss meat loaf or breaded something or other because they don't have bread crumbs. Walk into a health food store, buy a loaf of gluten-free bread—even if you don't like the bread—thaw it out, toast or break it up, and you have bread crumbs. You can choose from half a dozen loaves and make your own bread crumbs.*

5. *Build a repertoire of gluten-free products. Spices, soups, special dishes.*

You can't expect to do it right the first, second, or third time. You can't expect to know everything within the first or second month. There's a learning curve to it. And since it's a lifetime diet change, be patient with it. (George and Ceil Chookosian, owners, chef, taste testers, Foods by George)

21

Eating in the Real World

Right now it's easier for me to just eat at home. I used to love going out. I don't like having to repeat the same thing to the waiter and waitresses in front of my friends. They shake their head, listen, and then say: "Do you want pasta on the side?" (Linda, 62)

Anyone on a restricted diet knows that eating in is often easier and safer than eating out: the operative word is *control*. In fact, navigating real world dining can be initially daunting. There are always issues like cross contamination, the possibility of hidden sources of gluten when someone else is cooking, or that surprise birthday party when cake is served. Even the most well-meaning cook can render an entire platter of food inedible for someone with celiac disease by adding those last garnishes of parmesan toast.

Whether you eat out infrequently or with abandon, there are some good tips you should have in your toolbox.

One foolproof way around real world food is to **ask for unadorned food.** The concept is simple and straightforward. It is also easy to understand if your waitperson is challenged by the concept of gluten-free.

The description will grab the attention of the most jaded or confused waitperson, host, caterer, or chef. You can then ask for their help in getting you a safe and tasty meal. Don't be shy; be specific.

Over the years, I have learned that different approaches work for different situations. When I was first diagnosed and ventured out, I patiently explained that I could not eat any foods or products, additives, etc., with any wheat, rye, or barley in or on them. No bread,

*breading, flour, pasta. "Ah"—the waiter nodded understandingly—
"you're on Atkins!"*

*I then tried: I have a bad wheat allergy and can become ex-
tremely and immediately ill if I eat any food or product, additive, etc.,
with wheat in or on it. This tends to work—as much because many
restaurants will do anything necessary to keep you alive long enough
to pay the bill.*

*I use cards with the basics written on them translated into differ-
ent languages when traveling. This usually goes back to the chef—
many of whom are very responsive. Some come out to ask questions
and creatively work with safe ingredients; others send broiled salmon
or chicken breast with steamed vegetables.*

*I think that both the recognition and perception of celiac dis-
ease and gluten is changing and growing—because people keep
working at it.* (Rory Jones)

Learning how to eat in the real world is an important issue that is
getting easier by the month as celiac disease becomes more well known.
And the more they hear from customers, friends, relatives, and professionals about celiac disease, the more others will want to accommodate
the large percentage of the population that cannot eat gluten.

Conversely, only an ostrich with its head in the sand would say that
eating in the real world with celiac disease is easy. Whether you live to
eat—and feel terribly pinched by the diet—or eat to live—and happily focus on the company over the food—you must learn some basic techniques.

Restaurants

*There's a thin line between being obnoxious and being too shy or
nervous with a waiter.* (Mary, 50)

*We were in a French restaurant and the waiter kept going to the
kitchen and coming back. He finally told me: "The chef said he was
a chef, not a doctor."* (Michael, 42)

Restaurants, like people with celiac disease, come with different ethnicities and attitudes. But there is a great deal of common ground when
approaching them.

Restaurant dining requires the following:

- A knowledge of gluten
- A knowledge of restaurant practices
- A knowledge of specific ethnic food preparation
- An understanding of what questions to ask
- Perseverance

After you have mastered basic gluten (grains, ingredients, labels, and your own kitchen), it is time to master restaurant practices. Dealing with cross contamination (what is "on" the food, not necessarily "in" it) is the big issue, with preparation a close second.

If you have visited or worked in a restaurant kitchen, you learn that the better the restaurant, the safer (generally) the meal. The most sophisticated (i.e., expensive) kitchens have segregated work areas for desserts, vegetables, meats, sauces, frying, etc. The master chef puts it all together and "plates" it. Cutting boards are more segregated (i.e., less cross contaminated) and washed regularly. But this is not where most people eat when they go out. Therefore, it is important to understand how food is made where you regularly go and cultivate their attention.

I never liked cooking—we went to my mom's once a week, had pizza once a week, Chinese food once a week. Celiac disease made it hard. There's been an effect on our friends—they want to go to interesting ethnic restaurants. We cramp their style a little bit. (Jean, 54)

Using Personal Technology to Help Detect Gluten

When eating out it is reassuring to know that the food you are putting in your mouth is actually gluten-free. The good news is that there are now gluten sensors to help you test a food before you eat it. The not-so-good news is they are expensive, they can give false positives (alerting for gluten in a food when it is actually below the FDA-approved level) as well as false negatives (indicating no gluten when the food actually has some), and some are complicated to use. The most portable and restaurant-friendly of the devices/kits is the Nima.

The Nima Device

I love the Nima, but it is expensive. The device can generate errors that result in needing to retest and that five-dollar capsule is wasted.

This just adds to the already high financial costs of eating gluten-free.

I was getting persistently high antibody levels despite the fact that I thought I was eating gluten-free. I went back and thought carefully about where I was eating while at work and then I tested the items. It turns out places that claimed to be gluten-free were not and when I stopped eating at these places I felt much better and my antibodies (and biopsy) are looking very good.

Overall, I think it is an incredibly useful tool to set up your gluten-free eating in places where you cannot control your intake as easily (i.e., while at work or school or to test that go-to place that claims to be gluten-free) or when you have a language or cultural barrier. But I think one can use it sparingly and use it to help stay healthy. (Tom, 45)

The Nima is an antibody-based, rechargeable portable device that can be used to test small amounts of a given food. Most find that it is easy to use and the results are easy to interpret. There has been some difficulty in closing the instrument and the company now supplies a small wrench to help fasten the instrument.

A one-time-use disposable capsule is filled with a pea-sized sample of food. The lid is twisted and chemicals mix with the food and results light up on a display. It will show either a smiley face indicating that either no gluten or gluten levels below 20 ppm were found in the sample or a wheat icon and the text "gluten found." It does not behave all that well when values are around the borderline value of 20 ppm—it may record as "positive" values below this level (defined as gluten-free).

If you have a full plate of food, or several courses, every item must be tested separately using separate five-dollar capsules. The test does not guarantee that your entire plate of food is gluten-free. It also cannot test soy sauce, alcohol, pure vinegar, or beer, which is pointed out in the instructions.

Results from the Nima device can be sent back to the company, allowing for crowdsourcing data to be accumulated. We have analyzed this data and found that pizza and pasta were the foods that most frequently tested positive. Data also showed that 30 percent of food designated as gluten-free and tested by the device was positive. This rather astounding percentage reflects the difficulty in eating out for those with celiac disease.

The Nima is not meant to offer complete assurance that the meal in front of you is gluten-free. It is only meant to help in the decisions everyone with celiac disease must make. Nevertheless, it allows individuals to exert some control while eating out or even in the home.

There are other food sensors that will come to the marketplace in the future. While the Nima device is currently the only portable one, it is a step in the right direction. It should not be the only criteria patients use in restaurants and when eating out to ensure that their meal is safe.

There are also professional-grade test kits available to test for gluten. Test kits are a developing area in food technology.

"Back-Home" Techniques

Specific cuisines are made following tried-and-true techniques—often adapted to an American palate. Nevertheless, understanding the old-world methods will teach you a great deal about any given menu. If you understand how the cuisine is made "back home," it is easier to know what questions to ask and what to essentially avoid. If you love French food, pick up a good French cookbook and check how the sauces and dishes are supposed to be made. The same applies to other cuisines. This should enable you to ask appropriate questions and know which dishes may be problematic. Remember: no two chefs make a dish the same way, and there are many ethnic cuisines to explore.

Eating out was difficult at first. I used to eat out a lot. I went out the first time with my boyfriend and must have asked a million questions. I figured, what can they do to broiled scallops? The waiter said they would be okay, the vegetables would be plain, and I ordered a plain baked potato. Well, the scallops were on half a piece of French bread when they came out! Now, I try to call ahead. . . . I try to go to places I know are accommodating. (Lori, 31)

A Brief Sauce Primer

Sauces, as Julia Child taught a generation of Americans, are the "splendor and glory" of the art of French cooking. And they are made, almost uniformly, with butter and flour cooked together, the traditional roux, or last-minute beurre manié, which is butter and flour added to "finish" a dish.

Sauces are a major gluten source in most restaurants. Many French sauces are also routinely used in Continental and American cuisine, and even found in Greek moussaka.

Hollandaise sauce is made with eggs, water, lemon juice, and butter. Ostensibly safe. But restaurants may beat a tablespoon of béchamel or velouté sauce—made with flour—or a teaspoon of cornstarch (safe) into the egg yolks to "hold" a sauce that they need to keep warm for a long period of time. It is one of the tricks of the trade.

While reduction sauces should be safe, check with the kitchen. When in doubt, eat your food with sauce on the side.

RESTAURANT GUIDELINES

1. Ask to eat unadorned food and be ready with information on exactly what that means.

2. Read ethnic cookbooks. Learn about the ethnic cuisine(s) you like best and how your favorite dishes are prepared. Ask questions to make sure they are safe.

3. Understand restaurant practices (by cuisine, if necessary) to avoid cross contamination. This includes shared oil pots, cutting boards, garnishes, fried ingredients added to salads and dishes, sauce thickeners, marinades, prepreparation.

4. If you eat out regularly, frequent a few favorites and develop a good rapport with the owner/chef/headwaiter. Go there with your friends—more customers. Work with them to develop dishes you would like to eat.

5. The Internet has various sites that cover the cities you live in or will be traveling to that have good suggestions for gluten-friendly restaurants.

6. If you are returning food to the kitchen, make a small cut in it so that it is recognizable if it returns to you on another plate without the offending garnish or sauce.

7. Do not confuse every intestinal "burp" with gluten ingestion when eating out. People tend to eat food with a higher fat content and with more fiber when they are eating out. Multiple courses—with high-fiber fruit and high-fat ice cream to end—may be more food than you normally eat at a given meal. All this will affect the intestines.

8. Keep a positive attitude and persevere.

Other People's Homes

I tell people what I can and cannot eat. Wherever I go and I'm eating, I bring a bag of things I can eat. Anything I'm not sure of, I leave. (Fred, 63)

I always go into the kitchen at people's houses. (Mary, 50)

My friends are great. Some of my friends have stocked rice pastas and gluten-free food for me. When I go to a dinner party at a friend's house, I read labels. (Lori, 31)

If I'm not sure, I say no thanks, I'm not sure if I can have it. (Macie, 9)

A lot of times, I take my food with me—it's easier. I feel that I'm not imposing. (Linda, 62)

One of the most difficult real world eating situations is going to someone's house for dinner or a party. The home may be that of your best friend, an acquaintance, your boss, or your mother-in-law. Same food restrictions, different etiquette. A great deal depends on how well you know the individual, your own acceptance of the gluten-free diet, and your comfort level. If you go to the dinner party for the company, it is easier to maneuver the meal. This is an arena where people who are going to cheat often fall off the gluten-free diet rather than offend.

Eating disorders, diets, and food fads have transformed the eating landscape—everyone knows someone with a "food issue." Some are tolerant and others annoyed at the necessary accommodations. If the occasion is mandatory (see Chapter 22), taking the time to work out details beforehand is worthwhile. And carry backup supplies—just in case.

Warning a host(ess) is the best etiquette—you have to assume that no one wants either a miserable or sick guest.

If all else fails, and you are still uncomfortable eating out, start entertaining! Show your family and friends how it should be done.

GUIDELINES FOR OTHER HOMES

1. Call ahead. Ask what they are planning to serve.

2. Explain that you need plain food—and what that means.

3. Offer to bring something. A food allergy or intolerance provides you with a good excuse to bring some safe food so that you will not offend the chef. You might want to bring a doggie bag of gluten-free food to tide you over.

4. Snack or eat before you go. It is never a good idea to arrive starving for cocktail hour—whether or not you have celiac disease.

5. Examine the food being offered and find something safe.

6. If the dinner/event is catered, talk to the caterer. They may be able to give you something unsauced or made specially.

Hospital Stays

Logic dictates that it should be easy to obtain gluten-free food during a hospital stay—medical professionals should understand both the disease and the necessary dietary restrictions. This is not always the case.

During my pregnancy, my son had a high heart rate so I was in the hospital (at thirty-one weeks) for five days. I didn't have choices for meals, and there was nothing I could eat. I had the nutritionist in my room on a daily basis. For breakfast, they gave me regular (non-gluten-free) Rice Krispies, and I got the nutritionist back, who said: "This is what we give all of our patients with gluten intolerance." I showed him the box and showed him the ingredients (with gluten). It didn't matter. I told them, "I'm hungry, I'm pregnant, you're killing me!"

They got my son's heart rate stabilized and I went home. I was able to deliver when things were good at thirty-seven weeks. In the hospital, after I delivered, I would get food at mealtimes and I couldn't eat anything on the plate. I said: "What can you send me?" They sent nothing—told me the kitchen was closed. I had nothing for breakfast or lunch for two days. I was living on snacks and food delivered by friends in the celiac community. My husband was so busy (at work and taking care of my daughter at home), he could only come at dinnertime with food for me.

We talked to the head of nutrition . . . and the next day, I got a baked potato. It didn't make any difference. I quickly learned I couldn't depend on that. I wasn't getting any sleep. I wasn't getting any food. I finally broke down and asked to be sent home. My son had to stay in the hospital and I would come every day—with my own food—to be with him. (Alison, 34)

Conversely, one woman from the Boston area had a very different experience.

I contacted the hospital a week or two before I was due to deliver. I spoke to the nutritionist, who was very familiar with celiac disease and the gluten-free diet. The hospital actually had a gluten-free menu! To be on the safe side the nutritionist advised me to bring my own gluten-free snacks and told me there would be a microwave and refrigerator on the floor that I could use. The nutritionist gave me her pager number so that I could contact her when I was in the hospital.

When I registered at the hospital, they asked if I had any allergies. I told them I had a gluten allergy (even though that isn't what it is), so that everyone who saw me would see right on my chart that I had to be on a gluten-free diet.

Some of the foods on the gluten-free menu included French toast, chicken, turkey, fresh fruit, rice cakes, yogurt, omelet, rice, steamed vegetables, and salad. I didn't even eat anything I brought with me. The nutritionist came to visit me although I hadn't paged her. She had been notified I was there and just showed up. It was a very positive gluten-free hospital experience! (Trudy, 28)

If you are in the hospital on a nonemergency basis, call ahead and speak to the nutritionist to find out what arrangements can be made. If the hospital is not celiac-savvy, talk with your doctor and enlist his or her help. Bring supplies as if you were traveling. In an emergency, have a friend or family member advocate for you to obtain or bring in safe food.

This is one aspect of professional education that is slowly being addressed throughout the United States and will require personal diligence. Unfortunately, right now hospital food is almost as inconsistent as that found on many airlines.

Travel

I go to a lot of meetings. I send ahead and tell them I'm celiac and I get a special meal. I'm out of the country at least four times a year, in addition to my travel in the United States.

My general approach to airlines is to order fruit. If it turns out to be fresh cut, I eat it, and if not, I don't. And I always have something to eat with me.

I was just at a meeting in Sweden last week and someone from the kitchen came out. I find anywhere in Europe is great. They were much more sensitized. People were overly nice. (David, 51)

Travel adds an element of the unknown that many people with celiac disease initially find unsettling. They are afraid to leave the comfort and food-related safety of home. Those who must travel for business take the leap out of necessity. Whatever the reason, celiac disease should not stand in the way of "trains, planes, and automobiles."

The skills required for enjoyable travel are mainly about preplanning. Celiac disease will have the most impact on those for whom travel means strapping on a backpack, buying a rail pass, or renting a car and taking off. For those who have a wanderlust but are willing to take the time to research locations, restaurants, and local support groups and to carry enough emergency gluten-free food supplies for a few days of acclimation, traveling can regain some "normalcy."

We're not traveling as much. It is such a burden to worry about the food. It's easier not to go. I feel my children are missing a lot of travel opportunities. But we loved Disney World. Every chef knew about it (celiac disease) and was trained in it and didn't laugh at it.

They had gluten-free soy sauce in the Japanese/Polynesian restaurants. Never in my life was I so impressed. (Ilyssa, 33)

Some choose to travel on gluten-free trips and cruises that are available; others book commercial tours, travel with family and friends, or go solo. Whatever your choices, you must think about each aspect of your journey.

Where Are You Going?

Do you speak the language? If not, you will need a card explaining celiac disease and your eating requirements. Do not use one that claims instant crisis/collapse at the table if you ingest gluten. Many overseas restaurants will view you as more of a threat than a valued customer.

Does the country understand/have a celiac population? If so, making dining and hotel arrangements will be easier. Research local celiac organizations and find restaurants that are recommended.

Because of the cuisine, some parts of the world will be more difficult than others. But that should not hold you back.

I was diagnosed with celiac disease forty years ago. We've been to China, Russia, Morocco, Eastern Europe, Scandinavia, Australia, and New Zealand. Eastern Europe and Russia were the most difficult because everything had sauces. I would eat salad or plain potatoes. I always took frozen bread with me from the United States and rice cakes, peanut butter, nuts, and dried fruit.

I knew going to China was going to be hard—in many ways. I ate a lot of plain rice and steamed vegetables. I'm not one to make a scene. I think I lost five pounds on the trip. But it was wonderful. I'd love to go back. I loved the people. I went there to get a new experience, learn about the country and the culture. Food was a minor part of my travel. (Lou)

Transportation

Airline travel is usually about long lines, high security, and high anxiety. Trying to eat gluten-free on an airplane only heightens the tension. Many airlines offer gluten-free meals, but only some of them currently understand what that actually means.

Order a special meal but carry supplies that will take you to your destination. Bring "real" food on the plane with you. If you bring only trail mix and fruit on a very long flight, you may begin to feel like a squirrel. Pack a small insulated bag with an ice pack and layer it with several plastic bags filled with frozen chicken pieces, cheese, and any other cold food you like. The frozen food will slowly defrost, enabling you to eat safely for many hours on the go. Place it on the floor of the plane, which becomes and stays cold at thirty-five thousand feet. Vegetable sticks, fruit, and other nonperishables can go in a separate carry bag.

Make sure you have a bag of snacks and some of your gluten-free stash on the plane. Luggage does not always arrive or leave with its owner.

Prepare for delays in both arrival and departure at all connections. Airport food is uniformly gluten-filled. You may find yourself living on bananas and bottled water for twenty-four to forty-eight hours if you do not come prepared for delays.

Accommodations

The better the hotel, the more accommodating the management. If you can arrange for a room with a refrigerator, you can be assured of milk for cereal in the morning and a place for other perishable gluten-free items.

The hotel concierge should be able to help you find local stores to buy milk, juice, bottled water, fresh fruit, cheese, and other edibles. In Italy, for example, the local pharmacies carry gluten-free pasta, crackers, and snacks. Stock up; they are excellent.

Length of Stay

If you are traveling for an extended period of time—or through multiple locations—you should have ample dry supplies as well as the ability to replenish your gluten-free food needs in various locations. But you must preplan with either your tour director, travel agent, or various hotels in order to be assured of finding what you need when you need it.

Restaurants

Do research before you go and find at least one or two suggested gluten-free or celiac disease–friendly restaurants in every city you will visit. If necessary, go to these places more than once. Family-owned restaurants are usually very accommodating. Go early, before they get crowded.

If you plan ahead, bring lots of gluten-free food, and expect very little of the airline food, you may be pleasantly surprised to find many of your anxieties and expectations to be false. Fresh, safe, and delicious food is available throughout the world for the people traveling with celiac disease who are willing to seek it out. You may find yourself returning with most of your stash of gluten-free food.

I feel that I have no restrictions. Whether it be sports or traveling or going out to dinner or going to a wedding or whatever. There are ways you can deal with it. It's not traumatic or the end of the world. (David, 51)

Eating gluten-free in the real world can be frustrating. Practice may not make it perfect, but it will make it worthwhile.

22

Family Occasions

A crust eaten in peace is better than a banquet partaken in anxiety.

—Aesop

Holidays and special occasions add new meaning to eating in the real world. This is when your family and friends are loosening their own dietary resolve. Repeated urging to have "just a bite" of Grandma's lasagna, Mom's matzo balls, your sister's Christmas pudding, or your best friend's wedding cake underscores the implied assumption: this is no time to be "dieting." Interestingly, it is here that you can teach your family and friends who are dieting for other reasons how to turn a restriction into an attainable goal—with enjoyment and humor.

Holidays—Dealing with the Urge to Splurge

Holidays and festive occasions revolve around tradition and food. Easter, Passover, Thanksgiving, Christmas, weddings, confirmations, bar mitzvahs, funerals—everyone is expected to join in at the buffet, the table, and the bar. Toasts, roasts, and cake. In some families, not eating is tantamount to challenging tradition.

> *My mother thinks I've made the whole thing up to annoy her. My sister is a diabetic, and my mother thinks that's psychological as well. She insists on making the turkey with sourdough bread stuffing and puts bread crumbs on the string beans. I'm thinking of not showing up next year.* (Anonymous, 38)

When looking to the holidays, adapt what you can, bring substitutes for the whole family to sample with hints to incorporate them in next year's celebration, and focus on the holiday and the nonfood tradition.

Most of the foods served at the holidays can be readily altered to be gluten-free. The biggest hurdle may be convincing a sister or mother-in-law to make the turkey stuffing separately, if they insist on making it with gluten.

Nutritionists and medical professionals have long urged holiday celebrants to party "lightly"—including both food and alcohol. One of the biggest problems is actually the loss of inhibitions after several drinks and the tendency many people have to overeat or cheat on a diet "just this once." This is often the bigger issue for someone with celiac disease.

The actual foods that compose the major holiday fare—eggs, turkey, sweet potatoes, fresh ham, brisket of beef, chicken, nuts, dried fruits, cream, etc.—start out gluten-free. The basics are not the problem. Preparation and temptation can make them dangerous for someone with celiac disease, though. And both of these can be avoided with some advance planning and the right attitude.

Banquets and Wedding Bell Blues

Buffets, serving stations, and plated meals present an obstacle course of potential cross contamination. You may know what is in a salad or vegetable dish, but not how it has been handled, or how often a neighboring spoon sitting in pasta/gluten has dipped into it.

The best part of large parties is the variety of food served. While hors d'oeuvres often contain gluten, there are usually multiple courses later on that will offer enough to eat.

It's not the end of the world if you can't eat at a wedding. Concentrate not on what you can't eat, but on what you can. (Betty, 61)

Dieters of all varieties have the most trouble during holidays and festive occasions. People with celiac disease are not alone. The urge to splurge can undermine the most determined.

PARTY PLANNING

1. Call ahead. Talk to the caterer or banquet hall, find out what is being served, and determine the best way to handle the meal. Explain that you need gluten-free food and ask how you can work with them to accommodate those needs.

2. Snack ahead of time so that you are not so starved or alcohol driven by mealtime that you start to think about "just one bite."

3. Arrive at the buffet table early to get fresh dishes that have not seen spoon swapping.

4. Ask for a special meal if everything is pre-plated.

5. Mind your fats and sugars as well as your gluten.

6. Enjoy the occasion. Wedding cake usually looks better than it tastes.

23

The Medicine Cabinet and Cosmetics

Potations pottle deep.

−William Shakespeare, Othello

When first diagnosed, most people with celiac disease focus on the kitchen. It is equally important that they also focus on their medicine and cosmetic cabinets. Daily vitamins and drugs are often the culprit in nonresponsive patients who think that they are carefully following a gluten-free diet.

Prescription Drugs

Pharmaceuticals (prescription drugs) are made up of two basic components:

1. "Active" ingredients—the substances supplied in specific doses that act on your body to alleviate or target an illness or condition
2. "Inactive" ingredients—the substances that bind, cover, and help deliver the active ingredients into the body

"Starch" is a universal binder that is found on many prescription drug information sheets.

When examining drug labels, if the inactive ingredients are not listed, ask the pharmacist or your doctor to look them up in the *Physicians' Desk Reference* (*PDR*). The *Physicians' Desk Reference* contains a list of all pharmaceutical drugs detailing both the active and inactive ingredients. The pharmacist can also print out a full report of prescription drug specifications (they should come with the package) for you to examine.

By law, the basic "food starch" found in food is corn. The same regulations do not apply to prescription drugs. So while most drug manufacturers do actually use cornstarch when a binder is required, if the label does not specify this, you must call or ask a knowledgeable pharmacist.

Most prescription drugs have an 800 number for the manufacturer, which will put you immediately in touch with a customer representative or chemist. These people know about allergens and, increasingly, are gluten-savvy. You will probably be told that to the best of their knowledge the starch is, or is not, corn-based. For legal reasons, that may be the best that you will hear. And it is most likely accurate.

If you are taking a prescription drug with a wheat-based inactive ingredient, talk with your physician about substitutes. If it is a new prescription, look it up in the *PDR*. There are also compounding pharmacies throughout the United States and online that custom-make gluten-free prescriptions for you.

Over-the-counter (OTC) drugs and compounds do not require a prescription. They must adhere to FDA guidelines, but you still need to scrutinize the labels for inactive ingredients that may contain gluten. Most OTC drug labels have an 800 number on the box as well. If you are unsure of the ingredient, do not take the drug until you make the call.

Vitamins, Minerals, and Other Supplements

They're a market, not a medicine. (Anne Lee, R.D.)

Vitamins are, by definition, required in trace amounts. There is no evidence that amounts greater than the "daily requirement" are beneficial to an individual. In fact, excess amounts of certain vitamins can be toxic. Well-known examples are vitamin A, which can cause a fatty liver; vitamin D, which can cause high calcium levels and kidney stones; and vitamin B_6, which can cause neurological problems. We recommend that patients with celiac disease consume a well-balanced, healthy diet. Pills should not replace food. Taking a daily multivitamin should not be harmful, though consuming megadoses may be.

Patients may have specific medical conditions that warrant supplements. These should be discussed with your doctor.

Whether scientifically required or not, most people take some type of daily vitamin supplement. Many take multiple pills. Therefore, this is an important area for diligence in label reading. If your diet is varied and dietician guided, vitamins may not be necessary.

Vitamins and supplements are covered under the new labeling law (see Chapter 19) even though prescription drugs are not. If you or your child takes vitamin and mineral supplements, keep in mind that "wheat-free" does not necessarily mean "gluten-free."

Other dietary supplements come in many unregulated shapes and sizes. They claim to take you through thick (dieters) and thin (body builders), fight flu, fight aging, build your immune system, improve your eyesight, and sharpen your memory. There is only one thing for people with celiac disease to remember—labels cannot be trusted; they can be dangerous to your health.

Dietary supplements are not medicines—even though they are often marketed for medical conditions. They are not government regulated, and studies have shown that anywhere from 0 to 200 percent of an active ingredient may be in a bottle. There is currently no assurance that you are getting what is on the label—and you are paying handsomely for the privilege. Several recent studies found soybeans, wheat, rice, walnuts, and Alexandrian senna, a powerful laxative, in various supplement products, but not on the label.

The lack of government oversight of the manufacturing of dietary supplements makes their use by people with celiac disease suspect. All types of supplements must be carefully checked, including:

- Teas
- Protein drinks
- Tablets
- "Juices" (e.g., drinks that are not pure juice)

Enzyme Supplements

> *People will do anything to eat gluten again. Reminds me of snake*
> *oil salesmen in the Old West.* (Betty, 61)

Researchers are actively working to find enzymes that digest the fragments of gluten that are toxic to people with celiac disease. (See Chapter 27.) Several enzymes are currently being rigorously tested to ensure that they do not create any allergic or immunological reaction in the body, since they are foreign proteins being introduced into the digestive tract.

Nevertheless, various over-the-counter supplements are already being actively marketed in carefully worded advertisements that make various claims about digesting gluten, healing the gut, and reducing inflammation. They state in very fine print at the bottom of labels and websites that the supplements are not intended to treat or cure diseases. And they advise people to take their products without the rigid testing of effectiveness that the FDA requires. There are currently no over-the-counter enzymes that digest gluten and it is unclear as to whether they are safe.

Most people with celiac disease are careful about the foods they put in their mouth. They should be equally careful—or even more careful—about over-the-counter supplements.

Wheatgrass

Wheatgrass is a common ingredient in a lot of herbal and vitamin supplements. Technically, it is in the wheat family—it is the portion of the plant before the grain head develops. Some people have taken the stand that it is safe for people with celiac disease because it is not the portion of the grain containing gluten.

The question of contamination remains. This particular wheat and chaff may be inseparable. We do not recommend that people with celiac disease consume either wheatgrass or barley grass. More research is needed to determine the manufacturing processes used and the safety of this ingredient.

Toothpaste

Most toothpaste is gluten-free. It is more of an issue for children who may ingest an unhealthy amount of fluoride. Check labels, particularly if you use toothpaste manufactured outside of the United States.

Cosmetics

Lipstick

Can I kiss my girlfriend if she's wearing lipstick that isn't gluten-free?
(Anonymous, 16)

Lipstick is the only cosmetic that people ingest, sometimes in huge quantities. It is one of the more profitable sides of the cosmetics industry because we regularly lick, kiss, or eat it off our lips; then we reapply it and go through the process again. Even children try it on when they dress up.

Lipstick comes in many colors and flavors and different formulations. In particular, the long-lasting formulas often contain wheat germ oil or other wheat-based products.

Lipstick is not considered a food product, and the labels are not regulated by the FDA. If you wear lipstick, spend some time on the phone with the manufacturer to make sure that it is gluten-free.

Kissing. People who wear lipstick can consume a fair amount of it. However, it is hard to believe that those who kiss lipsticked lips would be ingesting much gluten by this method.

Lotions and Potions

Gluten is absorbed only through the digestive tract. It is not absorbed through the skin. Unless you are ingesting your shampoo, skin lotions, creams, or makeup, they do not have to be gluten-free. If you have specific skin sensitivities to creams that contain gluten, you may need to consult a dermatologist or an allergist.

Many patients with celiac disease feel that they come to the diagnosis with an "advanced degree" in Bathroom 101. Make sure that the medicine and cosmetic cabinets are part of your gluten-free knowledge base.

24

Is Your Gluten-Free Diet Healthy?

Food was my main concern. I didn't know what to feed my child. At first it was just plain meat and potatoes. It was such pure food.
(Sue, 41)

Anyone with celiac disease is acutely aware of what they put into their mouths. And that puts them in a unique position to control the fats and sugars that put them at risk for other serious medical conditions. At first, many patients eat simple, pure, unadorned food simply because they do not know what else to eat. Without realizing it, they have mastered the essence of a healthy, gluten-free lifestyle.

Real, that is, unprocessed foods—meat, fish, fowl, fruits, vegetables, potatoes, rice, specific grains—are safe and healthy. Depending on preparation, they are also lower in fat and sugar than processed food. This last point is crucial to the long-term health of people with celiac disease because they are still susceptible to obesity, diabetes, hair loss, hypertension, high cholesterol, and the diseases that accompany aging. If, like most Americans, they are overeating and not exercising, the problems are compounded.

Most important, these issues are more of a concern for someone on a gluten-free diet.

Spare the Fat and Spoil the Cake?

In the absence of gluten, the universal binder, some gluten-free foods contain more fat and oils to hold ingredients together. Many manufacturers also claim this is crucial to make the products "taste better." In addition, after patients eliminate many of the "low-fat" foods from their daily diet because of gluten-filled ingredient lists, they may find themselves eating a higher level of fat per day than before.

Gluten-free food is also usually lower in the nutrients and fiber found in gluten-filled products. Wheat-based cereals and breads, for example, are routinely fortified with additional vitamins and minerals. They are naturally higher in fiber. When this fiber is eliminated from the diet, many people neglect to find substitutes.

Scientific studies have not examined the "health" of a standard gluten-free diet. But you must ensure that your own diet, and that of your children, meets high health standards. There is a rich assortment of alternatives available, and they need to be introduced and integrated into everyday habits.

Disordered Eating

I follow a strict gluten-free diet, but I kept getting bloated and some diarrhea. Someone said that lactose can cause diarrhea so I cut out all milk products and cheese and that helped. Oh, and all of a sudden I started getting rashes on my arms. Really unattractive. And I read that tomatoes and citrus can cause rashes so I cut those out. Oh, and I don't eat corn because, well, I don't think it agrees with me. There are articles on corn allergies. I have to cut out a lot more than just gluten now and I feel better. And I think overall it's a healthier diet—my husband disagrees but he's not the one with celiac disease. (Vicki, 45)

The focus on food as both cause and cure for celiac disease can lead to disordered eating habits. Often, avoiding one food leads patients into the belief that eliminating other foods will clear up diverse symptoms that may have no relation to celiac disease or food consumption. As one food after another is eliminated, eating disorders emerge. In some people, food restrictions become excessive. There is an increased association of celiac disease with anorexia nervosa, which is an extreme example of disordered eating.

The Internet and the local food "guru" are not necessarily the source of good information. People with celiac disease embarking on a gluten-free diet should not do so on their own but with the help of a dietician. This is especially important if foods other than gluten are avoided, as in a low-FODMAP diet (see FODMAPs, Chapter 16).

Eliminating different foods in the hope of treating various symptoms can be unhealthy when essential minerals and vitamins are absent from a person's diet. Many people are excluding nutrients that keep them out of the doctor's office, not in it. If you find yourself eliminating one food after another (gluten, corn, soy, dairy, fats, carbohydrates, etc.) we strongly recommend that you discuss your diet with your gastroenterologist and meet with a nutritionist, who can help you maintain a balanced and healthy diet.

Cholesterol/Triglycerides

Prior to diagnosis, the cholesterol level of most people with celiac disease is low. This occurs mainly because they are not properly absorbing fat and cholesterol in the small intestine. As the gut heals, the picture changes.

Fat intake rises. First, patients start absorbing fat and cholesterol into the body. Then they start eating standard gluten-free products that tend to be higher in fat and sugar to make them taste better.

Fiber drops. The gluten-free diet is naturally lower in fiber as people focus on rice and potatoes and eliminate grains with gluten.

A high-fiber diet is used to control high cholesterol/triglycerides because the fiber binds to the cholesterol and helps to eliminate it. So, **people with celiac disease are faced with a diet naturally devoid of fiber, laden with additional fats, and an intestinal tract that is now absorbing it.** It is not a desirable recipe.

Children at Risk

Lily started getting her milestones back slowly. She had every therapy under the sun, and within the first six months she got really fat. She always bellied up to the counter to eat. Whenever anyone ate, Lily was right there with you. She had this amazing appetite and got huge. (Sue, 41)

An early diagnosis of celiac disease may reverse bone loss and other health problems. But many children have already developed eating behaviors based on a "starvation mode"—i.e., where they cannot get enough to eat and are always hungry. Now, they are absorbing food, gaining weight, and eating foods that may not be healthy for them on a long-term basis. They may be at *increased risk* for ancillary problems.

It is crucial that all children and adults on a gluten-free diet do the following:

1. Add grains and beans, such as quinoa or chickpeas, that are high in fiber
2. Add more fruits and vegetables
3. Eat raw and "crunchy, cooked" vegetables, as well as foods with skin to get as much soluble fiber as possible
4. Eat foods that are not high in fat and sugar

While it is important to focus on removing gluten from your diet, it is equally important to eat healthy. Adding soluble fiber to your diet will not only help to lower cholesterol, it will add variety and nutrients to the diet. But be aware that while fiber is essential, too much too soon can create GI symptoms that mimic indigestion.

Add the fiber slowly and give your body time to adjust. Be consistent—fiber is needed every day.

We may have a population of individuals with celiac disease diagnosed twenty years ago who are facing issues like obesity, heart disease, and diabetes. (Anne Lee, R.D.)

A Spoonful of Flax

Flax is a low-carb, high-fiber, and highly nutritious seed with a light nutty taste. It is a teaspoon of nutritional "honey" that easily disappears into baked goods, salads, and many other recipes. In families where grains other than rice (see Appendix B) are looked on as alien beings, ground flax may be the secret ingredient to healthier eating.

Flaxseeds can be purchased whole or ground. They are available at most health food and grocery stores. While the whole seeds will keep better, they have a hard shell that will pass through the body mainly undigested. Grinding them into meal releases their full nutritional benefit, which is considerable.

Once the seeds are ground using a coffee or spice grinder—or purchased as meal—they should be refrigerated. Grinding releases the high oil content of the seed, which will go rancid over time if not properly stored. Packages of flax meal can also be frozen and smaller amounts kept in a shaker in the refrigerator to be sprinkled on food when needed.

Because of the high fiber content of flax, it is also advisable to start slowly. It can have a laxative effect on people with a sensitive bowel.

Flax meal can be baked into muffins or breads, added to recipes, or sprinkled on soups, salads, pastas, cereals, toasts, waffles, and yogurts. Small packets—similar to the gluten-free soy sauce packets many people carry on trips or to restaurants—are available for easy use.

While flaxseeds are advertised in some places as the answer to everything from high cholesterol to hot flashes and certain types of cancer, they are certainly a meaningful addition to a healthy gluten-free diet.

Adults at Risk

I found a restaurant making ribs with gluten-free barbecue sauce. Nirvana. Boy, were they good. I achieved a "personal best" in cholesterol and fat at dinner that night. We go there regularly now. I'm so good with this diet—I deserve to eat something I really miss. (Gene, 48)

It is common for people on a restrictive diet to feel that they are entitled to indulge themselves. This may be as a reward for "being good" or simply out of frustration at the limited menu they live with. And even those who are compliant often splurge on food that is "safe" for one set of restrictions and every bit as bad for them in other ways. Many feel justified in eating half of a box of gluten-free cookies because they did not "cheat with wheat" at a restaurant or family party. Or pampering themselves with a sixteen-ounce steak (gluten-free but high in cholesterol) or a large bar of gluten-free chocolate (high in sugar and butterfat) to "make up for" the breaded or sauced food they miss.

Some people live to eat, but people with celiac disease must eat properly to live well. Your long-term health will depend on your ability to understand and enjoy eating healthy as well as gluten-free.

PART V

LIVING WITH CELIAC DISEASE

The shoe that fits one person pinches another;
there is no recipe for living that suits all cases.

—Carl Jung

Whether you perceive celiac disease as a lifelong hurdle or merely a speed bump, it is essential to stay on a gluten-free track. It is equally important to learn how to enjoy the ride.

25

Dealing with Children and Young Adults Who Have Celiac Disease

You can see a lot by observing.

—Yogi Berra

When children develop a chronic illness, the landscape of their lives, and that of their families, changes. Daily routines and expectations must be altered. If the only change required to return to health is a gluten-free diet, most young children—especially those diagnosed before age five—initially adapt quite easily. This is all they know.

The adjustment is often harder for the parents, who may feel their child is being deprived. Older children and young adults may also have adjustment problems because of social pressure and eating patterns and preferences that are already developed.

Factors That Affect Successful Adaptation

A great deal of research has gone into identifying the factors that promote a successful adaptation to a chronic illness in children. They include:

- The ability of the child to take control
- The severity/prognosis/functional status of the condition
- Personal characteristics

- Empowering families
- Support groups

These factors play a fluctuating role throughout childhood and well into adulthood. They are particularly important for young children with celiac disease. Early training in the diet and self-empowerment are critical. While parents cannot necessarily change their children's personal characteristics, they can acknowledge and work with them to maximize an acceptance of the illness and the diet.

Parental Attitudes

I have enormous guilt in giving this disease to my daughter. (Anonymous, 36)

I've made it my mission to feed her well. (Ilyssa, 33)

Parents, family, friends, and teachers play a large role in children's perception of and adaptation to celiac disease. These individuals set the tone and become, in large part, the enabling force that teaches children how to cope with the condition for the rest of their lives. This includes teaching children the skills needed to maintain the diet when it becomes difficult—i.e., as they grow and become independent.

Also important, children—as well as adults—absorb as much observing the reactions of the key people around them as by anything said.

Feeding their children is one of the first and most important duties of parents. It is understandable that parents may be overly concerned, anxious, and protective. Based on our interviews, it is also apparent that some parents go into denial, which may be extreme: "This is not happening to my child, at least right now."

One mother was most upset about her teenager not being able to go to the pizza parlor. Well, what about if she can't have a baby when she gets older and what if she has diabetes?

Another woman had a daughter about to go to college and didn't want to test her because she felt it would be too much of a change or adjustment before she went to school. Her daughter wasn't having any symptoms. But it's like child abuse if you have this knowledge, how could you not? (Sue, 41)

On one hand, it is important that parents learn to let go and enable their children at an early age. Conversely, it is equally crucial that parents understand that celiac disease, whose only cure is a change in what you eat, is a significant medical condition with many potential complications. Ignoring or denying its importance is extremely shortsighted. Sometimes, it is the parents who must develop better coping skills.

But the attitude that is most important is that of the patients. And, this may change quite dramatically as children grow up.

The First Five (Birth to Five Years Old)

I was a head counselor at a day camp, with a three-year-old group, and one of the little girls had celiac disease. I remember thinking how difficult that was for her, but also thinking: "She doesn't know anything else." (Melanie, 22)

Most very young children diagnosed with celiac disease develop a different sense and definition of "normal." If gluten-free food is the only type children have ever tasted, this becomes the norm.

She has no recollection of pizza or cake, so she devours her (gluten-free) food and adores it. She loves her pizza, loves her cookies and her treats. I know the personalities of her friends and would not give them something gluten-free if they are going to complain. Or I give them marshmallows or something universal, like ice cream—something they can both have. (Ilyssa, 33)

There's lots of things for people who don't have celiac disease. There are like five thousand things. For us, there are two thousand things. We still have a lot. And I think there are better things and healthier things. (Macie, 9)

Under the age of five, a child's diet and habits are regularly controlled by parents. Celiac disease, however, may have a significant impact on the entire family. Eating routines, food choices, and health concerns change. The response of the entire family to this impact affects the child's ability to adapt to the condition. Young children follow the lead of parents and siblings, and it is here that the seeds of acceptance, compliance, and self-empowerment are sown.

Start good eating habits young. This is an age when healthy eating can and should become a lifelong habit.

Empower the child. Some children are naturally self-reliant; others require more encouragement to develop that trait. Teach by example as you explain to others what celiac disease and gluten-free eating entail.

Involve your children in the process of living gluten-free. Teach your children about the gluten-free diet and encourage them to learn more. Involve them in selecting, shopping for, and cooking gluten-free food.

Set up a positive family dynamic around food. That way, the kitchen works as smoothly as possible for everyone. "Yours," "mine," and "ours" take on new meaning when children must share specific food supplies. Other family members may worry: "What about me?" These concerns must be addressed.

Reach out. Talk with other parents of children with celiac disease and hear their ideas; explore support group options and activities.

Encourage compliance—and explain why it is important.

For children of this young age, gluten-free is "normal"—unless you make it otherwise.

Six Ups (Six to Eleven Years Old)

I know a lot of children who are babied by their parents. I've always taken a very active role. I was very much included; nothing was kept from me. At doctors' appointments they didn't just talk to my parents, they talked to me as well. My parents' positive influence made it easier for me to deal with it. They gave me the freedom and control that was appropriate for a nine-year-old. They were good role models in how to manage it emotionally. (Mel, 22, diabetes/celiac disease)

Once children enter school, the rules change. Peer pressure, teasing, school lunches, teachers, school personnel, playdates, parties, organized sports, and many other activities and factors come to the fore. Other children's eating habits are regularly on display.

Our study showed that some of the greatest difficulties in maintaining the diet occur at times of educational transition—from kindergarten to grade school, from grade school to high school, and from high school to college. And children of this age are encountering the first of those challenges. Children are exploring who and what they are, their personal strengths and abilities. They are typically argumentative, self-conscious, and/or showing off and trying out new roles. This is when "owning" the gluten-free diet becomes a reality, or an argument.

Give them more responsibilities for their own foods. And encourage them to interact with teachers and other parents on their own behalf. The more control they can exercise over what goes in their mouths, the more self-reliant they will become.

> *I learned that you might have to eat different foods at snack time at school. And I never care. The (gluten-free) food tastes good!* (Ryan, 6)

Make teachers and other parents aware of the dietary restrictions your child requires. Make school transitions easier by starting each school year with information and gluten-free food supplies where appropriate. This might include talking to the classroom teacher, nurse, principal, other parents, or coaches. Some parents are tempted to intervene and advocate regularly for their children with celiac disease. Taking over this role, even for shy children, will have long-term consequences.

Anticipate—and teach your children this skill as it relates to food supplies. Children are spontaneous by nature, and this is a wonderful trait that should not be squelched. Learn to draw the line between compulsive planning and thinking ahead.

You are not a celiac; you are a person who happens to have celiac disease. Celiac disease is not *who* a child is; it is a medical condition he or she happens to have. Other children, and adults, can be dismissive or even cruel in their treatment of people with chronic illnesses. Being comfortable in one's own skin is a trait that many people lose after their toddler years and regain only much later in life. It is worth reinforcing at all ages.

Everyone is different. Having to eat gluten-free food does make a child with celiac disease "different," but everyone is different in some way(s). This lesson becomes increasingly important as children enter their teen years.

Involve your child in support group activities.

> It's pretty fun actually—you get to go to all these picnics and meetings and meet new people with celiac. At meetings, my parents find out more about celiac and I get to hang out with the kids who have celiac. (Macie, 9)

Navigating School

504 Plan

Grade School

For a school child, the restrictions of a gluten-free diet involve far more than maneuvering through lunchtime and snacks. Staying gluten-free at school can stand in the way of a child's ability to enjoy as well as thrive in an academic environment. The good news is that there are regulations in place—Section 504 of the federally mandated Rehabilitation Act of 1973 and Title II of the Americans with Disabilities Act of 1990—that can help to ensure that your child's school will initiate and implement a plan tailored to his or her needs. A 504 plan allows students with celiac disease to receive "reasonable" dietary and activity accommodations so that they can participate fully at school and have the same experiences and opportunities as their peers.

It is up to parents to decide whether they need to apply for and obtain a 504 plan for their child or whether the school is able to meet their child's needs through more informal discussions and negotiations.

The 504 plan ensures that staff members who deal with a student with celiac disease receive training in the management of the condition.

This includes teachers, classroom assistants, substitute teachers, cafeteria workers, office staff, school nurses, or any other staff who have primary care of the student. And it covers classroom art projects, field trips, and extracurricular activities as well as cafeteria planning.

Accommodations cover a range of areas for grade school and include:

- Permitting students to bring food from home and/or access to a microwave to heat it
- Informing parents in advance of activities involving food—and the ability to supply gluten-free options or opt out of activities
- Permitting safe storage of meals/snacks in the nurse's office, pantry, or cafeteria cooler

University

New and different challenges face college and university students. The 504 plan by this time may include:

- Dorm room assignment with access to a kitchen or permission to use microwave and refrigerator in the room
- Reduced usage or ability to opt out of meal plans
- Gluten-free meals prepared and served separately in a safe area
- Gluten-free meals and snacks available during off-cafeteria hours (when many college students do their snacking and eating)

A full guide for obtaining and implementing a 504 accommodation is available from the Celiac Disease Center at Columbia as well as from national celiac disease support groups and online.

Twelve Ups (Twelve to Eighteen Years Old, Adolescents)

I was a freshman at celiac, and a freshman in high school.
(Danielle, 18)

Children who are entering puberty are encountering tremendous social pressure to belong. Teenagers are beginning to separate from their family and identify more with their peers. This is where being

different—whether through clothing, diet, or habits—is often difficult. Suddenly, the diet they have been on for so many years is a social
disadvantage. Or they may be newly diagnosed and now forced to
redefine themselves, just as that "self" is emerging.

Studies show that **adolescence is another major transition period
where most breaking of the diet occurs.** There is a change in routines,
a less-structured atmosphere, increased peer pressure, a change in
teacher attitudes, and less parental oversight.

Encourage anticipation. Teenage planning tends to be a contradiction
in terms. Nevertheless, gluten-free supplies should be available for
stuffing into a backpack or sports gear. Teens should become adept at
and comfortable with calling someone who is giving a party to ascertain what is being served. BYO (bring your own) takes on an expanded
meaning.

Stay well supplied. Teenage boys, in particular, can have huge appetites.
Make sure there are ample gluten-free supplies in the kitchen. Make
sure the supplies and snacks are healthy.

Your body, your health, your diet. Adolescents with a chronic illness
must buy into their own care. This may require persistence. Much like
open discussions of drinking, driving, and sex, gluten-free compliance
should be part of the dialogue. There are long-term ramifications to
noncompliance, and teens need good information to justify the restrictions on their eating.

People with few or no obvious symptoms have the hardest time
when it comes to long-term compliance. The adolescents must trust that
the diagnosis is correct because most people who have been on the diet
for an extended period of time do *not* experience symptoms when they
eat some gluten. Showing biopsy results to children is one method to
reinforce the validity of the diagnosis.

Finding the appropriate approach to convince teens—or adults—to
comply with a diet they feel they may not need can be difficult. For some
patients, and their families, this is an issue that may require professional
assistance. Support groups are also a good source of information and
age-appropriate forums.

Teens can be self-conscious about their weight, their skin, their shape, and everything else staring back from the mirror. Healthy, low-fat food lessons may be welcome at this point. Adolescents should attend medical education programs where and when appropriate.

Watch out for eating disorders. Food is an emotionally charged issue in many families. It is one way for teenagers to rebel and to control. Eating disorders are common in the United States. Teenagers with celiac disease need specific foods to stay healthy, more so than many other teens.

There are several issues to be considered. First, many people with celiac disease who have vomiting and diarrhea may initially be falsely diagnosed with an eating disorder. Second, a genuine eating disorder and celiac disease can coexist. The onset of celiac disease in a patient already diagnosed with anorexia nervosa could increase the medical complications associated with anorexia.

If the food relationship has been good prior to adolescence, it should weather the storm. If not, intervention may be necessary.

Adolescents with Celiac Disease and Type 1 Diabetes (IDDM)

Adolescents with a double diagnosis of celiac disease and type 1 diabetes must deal with two chronic illnesses and a host of health-related activities/restrictions. It is, without doubt, a large burden. You must not only adjust your insulin when everyone else is going for a slice of pizza—you must now also figure out what to eat in order to be part of the group.

The current practice in the United States is "carbohydrate counting." It is based on the theory that the foods that increase blood sugar the most are the carbs and, in order to regulate blood sugar and insulin units, patients must evaluate the number of carbs they eat per day and per meal.

The essence of carb counting is that a "one carb" serving (a slice of bread, a glass of milk, etc.) is the equivalent of 15 grams of carbohydrate.

Gluten-free products do not fit quite as neatly into the basic carb scenario. While one slice of whole wheat bread is approximately 15 grams of carb (or "one carb" count), one slice of gluten-free rice bread is approximately 18 to 20 grams of carb. This extends to

most of the gluten-free products (pasta, cereal, crackers, etc.). Over
the course of a day, the difference can be significant. Therefore, the
insulin must come up or the carbs must come down. The priority is
the amount of carbs, not the source. (Anne Lee, R.D.)

Insulin and Weight Control

Some adolescents learn to manipulate their insulin to manage weight control. As described in Chapter 12, insulin brings the glucose in food into the cells for use. If it is not absorbed into the cells, it is excreted in the urine. If there is a lack of insulin in the bloodstream (hyperglycemia), the body begins to break down fat to get the energy it requires. This, in turn, increases ketones in the bloodstream. This is the principle of the Atkins diet, though with diabetes, ketones are a signal of poor diabetic control.

The misuse of insulin dosage to manipulate weight may result in hyperglycemia and ketosis, which can cause patients to pass out and/or have other diabetic complications. It is particularly nutritionally dangerous for anyone with a dual diagnosis of type 1 diabetes and celiac disease.

Young Adults (College and Up)

In college everyone is very focused on their own world and their
own past and what they need to get done and where to go next; in
high school my friends were much more focused on me . . . they
knew me when I was diagnosed. In college, I didn't know anyone.
(Melanie, 22)

In college it takes a very strong person to do what's best for your-
self. (Roni)

Leaving the house—for college or the workplace—is a big transition. There is no gluten-free kitchen or food supply readily available at all hours, or an understanding family and group of old friends to turn to. And new schoolmates and coworkers may not understand celiac disease or what a gluten-free diet entails. People often hide their "illness" in order to be more readily accepted into the group.

A diagnosis of celiac disease, coming in college or young adulthood, can be an especially difficult adjustment. There is tremendous peer pressure to conform. Pizza, beer, bagels, and cereal may be diet mainstays out of necessity as well as choice. Nevertheless, the factors that affect successful adaptation remain the same as earlier in childhood. Coping skills come in all personalities and dimensions; they only require nurturing.

Call ahead. For any young adult heading toward college, the school, health center, and food services should be informed of the student's medical background and needs. Colleges will require advance notice, and a doctor's note, to allow a refrigerator and/or toaster oven in an individual room. These are important items to have ready access to.

Advocate for yourself. Learn to explain your needs and find the resources (restaurants, school cafeterias, snack bars, refrigerators, kitchens) to eat safely.

Taking charge. College students and young adults usually spend a great deal of time on the computer. They are capable, and should be encouraged, to order their own gluten-free food from websites and online stores. Parents can assist with ongoing support, good information, and, perhaps, containers with frozen and bagged emergency food delivered to the room or apartment freezer. The college should provide gluten-free dining options, but they may not be easily or uniformly accessible.

Keep a stash. Last-minute plans and busy schedules regularly destroy mealtimes. Since midnight pizza is no longer an option, keep and carry a stash of gluten-free food and snacks on hand to tide you over.

Eating nutritiously feeds the party animal. It is not always easy to eat well, or nutritiously, when on the run, but this should be a goal. Skin, hair, nails, physique, concentration—all improve on a healthy, well-balanced diet.

Although this is a time of great individuality and independence, reaching out to others with celiac disease is informative, beneficial, and comforting. Support groups and medical education seminars and conferences all supply important information on lifestyle as well as the diet and disease. They also usually have taste testing (i.e., free food).

I told my college friends: aside from getting a stomachache, now I'm worried five to ten years down the road, if I want to have a child. I don't want that to be another issue. I've sort of made that the important point to them. Celiac disease can cause serious problems if not dealt with properly. Once I said that, they got it properly. It is not just a stomachache: deal with it. (Melanie, 22)

Transition of care. There needs to be a transition of care from pediatrician to adult gastroenterologist as children grow up. These patients also should have access to their diagnostic records. We see many people who were given a very questionable diagnosis as a child when other family members were diagnosed. Unless the diagnosis was rigorously confirmed, it probably needs to be reestablished.

Road Rules

I told my daughter, "You now have the power to heal yourself." (Roni)

As children grow and develop, they need to steer their own course. In many ways, dealing with celiac disease is like learning to drive:

1. Teach them the road rules.
2. Teach them to *always* navigate a safe course.
3. Remind them to look every which way at crossings, and observe caution at the speed bumps.
4. Encourage and empower them to be patient with other reckless and rude drivers.
5. Give them the keys when they want to take a test spin. Experience and self-confidence make the best drivers.

26

Adults: Coping with Change

The division point between those who go on to lead a good life, no matter what the disease may be, and those who do not is accepting that your life has changed. It is a process of evolution. You must decide to live your life as well as it can be, given this change. There definitely can be a grieving process—tears and anger can be normal. No one can talk you out of that period. But there has to come a point where you close the door on life as it was—and go forward with life as it is. (Sue Goldstein, founder of the Westchester Celiac Sprue Support Group)

The patient leaves the doctor's office with a diagnosis: celiac disease. The prescription is a gluten-free diet. Unfortunately, compliance with a life-long gluten-free diet is sometimes easier to prescribe than to swallow.

Reactions to the Diagnosis

The psychological reactions to the diagnosis vary in both range and intensity. They may include a variety of feelings:

- Loss of control. My body has betrayed me and I am no longer in charge of my health.
- Mourning/loss. I can no longer eat whatever and whenever I want to. Some people actually mourn the loss of favorite foods.
- Insecurity. What will this mean and how will I ever learn enough about the diet to be safe? How will my family/boss/friends react?
- Anger. Why me?

- Denial. Why is a complete change in diet and lifestyle required to treat "silent" symptoms?
- Disbelief. Other doctors could not figure this out. Maybe the doctor is wrong.
- Resistance. I cannot/will not deal with this right now.
- Acceptance. Years of painful symptoms are suddenly explained, and people are "thrilled," "relieved," "grateful," that the "cure" is a diet, not a painful procedure or course of drugs.

I said I don't care as long as it's not a malignancy—I'll deal with it.
(Elaine, 55)

Whatever the initial reaction, a diagnosis of celiac disease means one thing to all: there will be change in their lives.

Dealing with "Forbidden Fruit"

Numerous studies of patients with chronic illnesses that require dietary and/or lifestyle restrictions have been conducted. The studies mainly examined diabetics, but also included patients with asthma, heart disease, epilepsy, celiac disease, and kidney failure. An analysis of the studies on celiac disease demonstrates that anywhere from 20 percent to 80 percent of patients consistently adhere to the diet.

There are many factors that influence adherence to a restricted dietary and/or lifestyle regimen. These include:

How—and What—You Are Told

Arguably, the most important factor affecting patients' adjustment to celiac disease is the way they are launched into the gluten-free world. Patients walk out of the doctors' offices with an attitude about the disease that may influence their state of mind for months to come. This includes not only how they are told, but the support offered by doctors and their staffs.

Patients left to fend for themselves may be overwhelmed by the gluten-free diet—a bad start even for those who are self-reliant. Patients guided toward knowledgeable nutritionists, support groups, and good medical and product information get a jump-start that makes the transition easier.

A study in 1997 showed that noncompliance with both lifestyle modification and medication regimens in chronic diseases is a major health problem. And that one of the most effective strategies for countering noncompliance was improved patient-physician communication.

How Sick You Were

I was never really as sick as other people are—no diarrhea, losing twenty pounds and sickly. It was, let's just do this test and see. So I think it was hard for me to initially see the benefit of the diet. I was just doing it with a grudge. Then I began to see the changes occurring with it. I certainly have more energy than I did a year ago. (Pete, 22)

Patients who suffered for many years with painful symptoms are usually the most relieved and compliant. The desire to get well is a powerful adaptor. They are usually pleased—even delighted—to embrace any changes that will heal them.

Those patients diagnosed with "silent" celiac disease tend to be less compliant. They did not feel badly to begin with and cannot always rationalize a restrictive diet on the basis of long-term complications—which may or may not occur. It is harder to change your life without the reward of feeling better.

Speed of Healing

Once you are on a gluten-free diet, improvement does not always occur on a rapid upward curve. Patients who are very sick prior to diagnosis may require additional drug therapy. They may be sick for an extended period of time, which may impact their reaction to a diet that is perceived as "not working." In some cases, they may be correct. Another problem—such as microscopic colitis, bacterial overgrowth, or underactive pancreatic function—may be responsible for symptoms not improving. When treated, these patients rapidly return to good health.

Your Coping Style(s)

I feel overwhelmed most of the time. I always have to prepare to go out, to travel. I'm always packing a food supply. (Pat, 45)

There are many people who think—How many times can I put my hands on the flame and not get burned? And you want that reaction, you want that sign to know. (Elaine, 55)

Some people, every little thing is very traumatic for them . . . hard to deal with. I'm just the opposite of that. I can deal with whatever cards are on my table. Even though I love the bread, I pass bakeries and just smell it. I'm very adaptable. I just say, okay, now I have this, how am I going to deal with it? It's just my nature . . . and some people don't have that. (David, 51)

A person's reaction to illness or any other trauma is determined by their individual style and coping skills. Some immediately take control of the diagnosis—as they approach most things in their life. They "dive in" and use mechanisms developed early in life that enable them to deal with adversity. These individuals tend to be:

- More flexible and adaptive to new and adverse situations
- More positive and proactive in their outlook
- Able to relax and laugh (at themselves as well as situations)
- More self-reliant

Others must develop these coping skills if they are to succeed at the diet and may initially find themselves out of control—of their body, their food, and their former lives. Familiar patterns established over a lifetime must be changed or eliminated, and the options may not be appealing. They find ingredient lists confusing, friends and family unsupportive, and the outside world threatening. A study of patient perception of the burden of celiac disease placed it second only to end-stage renal failure and need for dialysis.

Age, sex, and degree of illness also affect a person's ability to cope. People who were sick for many years before diagnosis, or who get sick after they ingest gluten, are usually the most compliant with the gluten-free diet. These patients have a tangible reward—feeling better—when in compliance.

Hypervigilance

I'm constantly on edge when we go out, even at a friend's house, worrying about a sauce or something lying on my food or touching it with flour on it. Cocktail parties are the worst—hors d'oeuvres are never gluten-free, even when the server says they are. I don't think

I've really relaxed at a party or eating out since being diagnosed ten years ago. (Vanessa, 54)

Hypervigilance is an enhanced state of sensory sensitivity to specific situations or activities that is accompanied by exaggerated behaviors. People with celiac disease who are hypervigilant are overly sensitive to their eating environment and constantly anticipating "danger" from unsafe foods. Examples of these hypervigilant behaviors include not eating out, taking your own food to events, and exhaustively grilling food servers. It is not a condition, but a way of behaving caused by the perceived need to maintain a strict gluten-free diet. It is important to know that extreme behaviors or hypervigilance can have negative consequences for someone on a gluten-free diet as they may bring about increased anxiety, fatigue, and an impaired quality of life.

Thus, while strict dietary adherence is encouraged, it may have adverse consequences. Importantly, parents of children with celiac disease need to teach adherence, not hypervigilance, which can lead to lifelong anxiety around eating. These hypervigilant behaviors are also associated with the development of eating disorders.

People with celiac disease who are on a gluten-free diet need to develop techniques that enhance adherence without taking a psychological toll. It is important to balance social and emotional well-being with informed, but sensible, dietary avoidance.

One can only be on a gluten-free diet, not a *very* gluten-free diet.

The Reaction of Family and Friends

The hardest thing is other people minimizing it. You don't have a wheelchair or a bald head, so people figure you're fine. (Perry, 53)

Studies show that dietary behavior appears to be particularly susceptible to social support and influences. Family and friends may minimize, distrust, or misunderstand the diagnosis. Reactions such as "it's only a food allergy" are incorrect, and "it could be so much worse" is not very comforting. It *could* be so much worse, but you may not be feeling well enough to think so. And you do actually have a serious medical condition that is being diminished in importance and relevance by those closest to you.

The reaction of spouses and significant others also plays a large role in patients' outlook and attitude. Interestingly, many men deny their illness and make the diet their spouse's problem. And the women work overtime to make their husband's diet gluten-free and to minimize its impact on his lifestyle. But the opposite does not always happen.

A number of single patients interviewed were concerned about the effect a gluten-free diet would have on their dating life. Several related similar stories of singles who either would not follow the diet or get tested.

> I'm forty-one years old, I'm divorced, I'm in the dating world. I want to go out on dates. I don't want to sit there with my date in a restaurant and be picky about what I'm going to eat. It's not a time in my life I want to deal with this. (Anonymous, 41)

Some family members may be embarrassed by the person with celiac disease who regularly questions waiters and friends before eating anything. Teenagers and young adults may actually resent this type of attention. Many younger siblings may be frightened: What does this mean for *me*? Will I get it? Will my food change? The tone of business lunches changes when one attendee acts so demanding.

Our studies on "partner burden" emphasize that a diagnosis of celiac disease has far-reaching effects on a family unit. Family and friends must adapt to the dietary and lifestyle changes as well as the patient. It is important to give everyone the information and time required to do it successfully.

The Support You Find

> The best thing I ever did was join a support group. I was so alone; the best thing was meeting other people going through what I was. I became active in the group and started helping others. It was my way of taking control back. I learned so much. (Heather, 43)

> I think the purpose of support groups is to give people the tools to get on with their lives. If you need some help, we're going to be there for you. And I think initially, the gluten-free diet takes a lot of getting used to.
>
> At first it's confusing because you're used to eating a bagel and cream cheese every morning and now you are told you can't. But the

majority of the people we talk to are absolutely thrilled that they finally know what's wrong with them after countless years of being sick.

A lot of people refer to themselves as "sufferers." Some people suffer for a long time . . . until they are diagnosed, and then the suffering is over. (Elaine Monarch, executive director/founder, Celiac Disease Foundation)

The gluten-free diet takes a lot of practice in order to acquire the skills and tools needed to feel comfortable in the real world. No one is an expert overnight. Support groups offer assistance in every aspect of the process. Meetings are often centered around medical speakers and present the opportunity to exchange information, stories, product news, resources, and problems with others who eat and live gluten-free. They also give people the chance to help those who are just starting out. Meetings offer the kind of encouragement needed to stay the course when frustration may lead to noncompliance or despair at ever getting it right. They can steer people to good resources on the disease, the diet, products, and stores available on the Internet. A word of advice: join a group where discussions are realistic and beneficial and focus on medical, dietary, and lifestyle issues of real import.

Some patients are adamant that they know everything about the diet—despite consistently positive test results. They often refuse to see a dietician or to join a support group. It is important to remember that knowledge of the diet is a continually evolving process. Do not stop learning.

Language Barriers

Finding support and obtaining gluten-free food can be difficult when there is a language barrier—as anyone who has traveled knows. Studies have shown that minorities had greater difficulty with compliance. The researchers noted in explanation that people in minority groups had more difficulty in obtaining sufficient information concerning the gluten-free diet.

Minorities also find it harder to read product labels written in an unfamiliar language. We have found this in the Hispanic population in New York. Some support groups are supplying Spanish-language translations of their material.

Medical professionals and support groups must be sensitive to those where language is a barrier to obtaining information and support.

Passing the Pizza Test

I always thought about food a lot. Now I think about it more.
(Mary, 50)

In all of our interviews, pizza stands out as the single most desired and "missed" food. The sight, smell, and anticipation of a pizza can literally make a person's mouth water. Patients describe eating the cheese off the one remaining piece in the box; walking past pizza parlors and smelling the aroma—but not going in; eating half a slice and getting sick; dreaming about it; successfully substituting gluten-free pizzas and enjoying them more and more; eating something else they really like instead.

Everyone has their own dietary "pizza"—and learning how to pass up these items is crucial to remaining compliant.

Helpful Hints

Find Ways of Rewarding Yourself

Find ways to gratify the urge to splurge without destroying the lining of your intestine! There are many delicious gluten-free foods. Explore your options.

Break Old Habits

Focus on what you *can* eat, rather than what you are missing.

Put Things in Perspective

Celiac disease is a serious medical condition, which has a dietary cure. Few serious illnesses have such a positive outcome.

Treat Yourself the Way You Treat Your Children with Celiac Disease

Many mothers (and fathers) with celiac disease take better care of their children with the condition than of themselves. Adults need to empower *themselves* and create their own success story. (And eat healthy meals.)

Let Go

The diagnosis of celiac disease alters the norm in an adult's life. Accept—and enjoy—those alterations and move on.

My priorities have changed. I think celiac disease made me focus more on what's important to me and let go of what's not. . . . Being celiac turned my life upside down for a while and changed it forever, but it's not the essence of who I am. (Heather, 43)

If you have to have any disease, this is a good one to have. All you have to do is stop eating the wrong foods and you're cured. It's not that difficult. (Fred, 63)

The gluten-free diet is a cure: few prescriptions are either that effective or tasty.

27

Research: Finding a Cure

The current "cure" for celiac disease is a gluten-free diet. However, researchers are actively pursuing alternative nondietary therapies. While most of the therapies are still in the early stages of development, several drugs have advanced as far as clinical trials. Drugs are being developed right now to help with the gluten-free diet. We hope that soon they will replace the diet.

There are several distinct reasons for this search for a cure that spring from both patients and medical communities. First, many patients want one. They have indicated that they find it hard to avoid gluten, and studies show that many patients cheat while on the diet, mainly in social settings. Our recent lifestyle study at the Center reported that 90 percent of respondents said that they strictly followed a gluten-free diet. Tellingly, in the same study 80 percent admitted that they cheated! A British study showed that 75 percent of patients with celiac disease ingested gluten, either knowingly or unintentionally.

In addition, follow-up intestinal biopsies do not always normalize in 30 percent of patients—an indication of ongoing gluten ingestion.

An understanding of the origin and physical basis of celiac disease has enabled researchers to see where the process and progression of celiac disease could be altered. Further research into the mechanisms underlying the response to gluten in susceptible individuals is the key to finding a satisfactory cure.

Potential Therapies

Potential therapies start at the top of the chain of events—gluten.

Genetically Modified Wheat

Currently, there is no GMO (genetically modified) wheat in the U.S. However, it may be possible to alter the grain—removing the toxic fragment—enabling people with celiac disease to eat wheat.

However, this is challenging because wheat is incredibly complex in its genetic makeup and the diversity of its immunogenic proteins. There is also a great deal of variety in the large number of different wheat types grown.

There are several potential lines of investigation. One is to identify types of wheat inherently lower in the amount of toxic gluten components. Another is to silence by "knocking out" (i.e., editing) some genes responsible for producing the toxic peptides or protein fractions.

While most research has been done on wheat, work is being done on other gluten-containing grains as well. There are several groups worldwide working to make gluten-containing grains nontoxic while maintaining their baking characteristics.

Another approach is to alter the gluten during breadmaking. The fermentation process used during the making of sourdough bread does eliminate some gluten but not enough to render the product gluten-free. Unfortunately, the process to create less gluten also makes the product less like bread and more like a cookie in studies performed in Italy.

Tight Juncture Regulators: Larazotide Acetate (INN-202)

It is known that the toxic gliadin molecule gets past the epithelial cells lining the villi into the *lamina propria* (part of the lining of the intestine beneath the surface cells) to trigger the immune response. (See Figure 3, page 12.) This occurs via at least two mechanisms. One is *between* the epithelial cells through the tight junctions that hold the cells together—and the other is *through* the epithelial cells. The relative role of these routes is unclear but both are part of a normal process that some have called leaky gut. In some people, these gliadin molecules that enter the lamina propria activate the processes that cause celiac disease.

Larazotide is a modulator of these tight junctions and appears to regulate them and partially block the passage of gluten through the intestinal barrier. Phase II testing, in which patients were randomly assigned to be given either gluten and a placebo or gluten and larazotide for a six-week period, showed a protective effect of the drug. It was generally well tolerated and effective against small amounts of gluten. Oral capsules were taken just before eating and worked for about two and a half to three hours. Those that received larazotide had fewer symptoms and fewer developed anti-tTG antibodies. A Phase III trial (see Drug Trials, page 284) is underway. Hopefully, more studies of this promising drug will be undertaken.

Oral Peptidases

Researchers are investigating enzymes (oral peptidases or glutenases) that digest the toxic fractions of gliadin. These fragments are resistant to digestion by the normal digestive enzymes in the intestinal lumen and are active in the acid-rich stomach. If the enzymes supplied as a medication could digest all these toxic fragments in the stomach, gluten would be safe to eat. Researchers have identified a number of different enzymes from diverse sources, including commercially available probiotics, fungi, and various bacteria and grains that can digest gluten.

A number of questions remain with this type of approach. First, it is known that less than 100 milligrams (mg) of gluten a day is sufficient to cause damage to the mucosa. Therefore, oral peptidases would have to digest, for example, 98 percent of the 3,000 to 4,000 mg of gluten present in one sandwich. This would require an extremely large amount of enzyme in order to prevent all of the gliadin fragments from getting through to the mucosa and provoking an immune response. Second, the enzyme would have to work in both the acid environment of the stomach and the more alkaline pH of the small intestine.

Most enzyme preparations being currently studied are to be used with a gluten-free diet when there is a limited amount of gluten contamination.

Latiglutenase is a combination of two enzymes that have been shown to be effective in breaking down the toxic components of gluten in the acid environment of the stomach. However, placebo-controlled studies in patients with celiac disease did not meet the planned primary endpoints of the studies as the study drug had the same effect as the placebo. However, there was a subgroup who did benefit from the drug. This provided enough impetus to allow for further studies of latiglutenase. Other enzyme preparations are being developed in both the U.S. and Europe. A powerful enzyme active against gliadin in the acid pH of the stomach has been developed by researchers at the University of

Washington. In addition, the glutenase preparation developed in the Netherlands has been released over-the-counter but has not undergone rigorous FDA testing to demonstrate if it is both effective and safe.

There are enzyme preparations that claim to digest gluten that are marketed as dietary supplements over-the-counter. They have a variety of disclaimers on the label such as "not sold to diagnose nor treat" anything. While they *imply* they have the ability to digest gluten, they have not undergone stringent FDA clearance processes to demonstrate safety and efficacy. (See Are They Safe?, below.)

Where Does the Treatment Fit In?

The currently developed medications, including larazotide acetate and enzyme preparations, are considered to help people with the gluten-free diet—not to replace it.

Should enzyme therapy be used as a supplement to the gluten-free diet? Since it is difficult to be 100 percent gluten-free, enzyme supplements or permeability blockers could be used to "cover" an occasional dietary lapse or cross contamination. Or will patients take a pill and eat whatever they wish? An interesting analogy is with cholesterol-lowering drugs. If patients take their cholesterol pill and then proceed to eat a cheese omelet with a side of bacon for lunch, and a large steak and potato stuffed with sour cream and cheddar cheese for dinner, they may "oversaturate" their medication. That is, the drug will not be able to handle/absorb the cholesterol load being digested. What then will be the immediate and long-term effects on a patient with celiac disease if they eat a gluten-filled diet and regularly oversaturate their enzyme pills? Many experts in celiac disease are concerned that the therapies will become a license to cheat, and the harmful effects of this will take decades to become obvious.

Are They Safe?

All medications carry the risk of side effects. Often this is not discovered until many thousands of patients have taken the drugs. The effect is not always apparent or identified in the more limited number of patients who take the drugs in clinical trials.

Enzyme therapies introduce foreign proteins from different organisms into the digestive process. They may potentially cause allergic—or other—reactions.

Oral peptidases and any of the proposed therapies offer exciting possibilities for the celiac community, but they also pose dilemmas that require extensive testing and research.

It is important that patients do not confuse the over-the-counter enzyme supplements currently advertised as "digesting gluten" with the oral peptidases being developed by various research groups in the U.S., Australia, and Europe. These various supplements are not tested according to FDA standards, indicated to treat celiac disease, or necessarily safe. They do NOT digest gluten.

Immunizations

There has been considerable research into inducing a tolerance to gluten through immunizations such as ImmusanT's Nezvax2 as well as nanoparticle therapy. There is precedence to this approach, since allergy shots also expose the immune system in a controlled way to induce tolerance as well as vaccines for various infections.

Researchers worked on a gluten peptide-based vaccine that might be used to desensitize or induce tolerance to gluten. The vaccine would be HLA-DQ gene–specific. It would target the sites where antibodies to gluten are produced and bind. While this is a very exciting direction of research, clinical trials were not successful as the vaccine supplied no more protection than the placebo. Perhaps a more broad range of peptides would have been beneficial, or even the entire gluten molecule, as in the nanoparticle therapy. However, it must be noted that with each clinical trial we learn so much more about the disease and how people react to the different therapies.

In Australia, researchers investigated treating people who have celiac disease with relatively benign intestinal parasites—a species of hookworm. This is another way of stimulating, or tricking, the intestinal immune system into developing protective immune responses. There has been work using this form of therapy for Crohn's disease and various allergies.

Lessons from the Vaccine Trial

While the vaccine trials were not successful, they resulted in many important lessons into the development of celiac disease in an individual. They revealed a new model of how T cells—those that trigger the immune response—are activated by gluten ingestion and cause symptoms in susceptible people.

We now understand that the reaction to gluten for those with celiac disease who are on a gluten-free diet is not "delayed"—it occurs upon ingestion and causes the release of the cytokine IL-2 (see Cytokine Blocker, page 282) that causes GI symptoms. The dominant symptoms are nausea and vomiting after one to two hours, not diarrhea or bloating. The latter symptoms are more likely to be from another component of the diet, possibly FODMAPs. (See FODMAPs, Chapter 16.)

Interestingly, this reaction also occurs in people with no symptoms prior to diagnosis—possibly found through screening relatives—who, after starting a gluten-free diet, experience severe symptoms with gluten exposure.

The elevation of IL-2 after the ingestion of gluten in those with celiac disease may become the basis of a new test. This could be used in those people with a sensitivity to gluten who went on a gluten-free diet prior to testing for celiac disease. After an oral gluten challenge, elevation of IL-2 after possibly one or two hours would confirm celiac disease as the cause of the gluten sensitivity.

Blocking Tissue Transglutaminase (tTG)

When the gliadin molecule gets into the lining of the intestine (lamina propria), it is acted upon (deamidated) and its chemical structure changed by the enzyme tissue transglutaminase. The deamidated gliadin fragment is then "primed" to interact with specific genetically driven receptors on specific cells, setting off the inflammatory response that results in the destruction of the villi. (For a more complete explanation of tTG deamidation and the genetic sequence, see A Genetic Primer—Fitting the Groove, Chapter 6.)

Researchers are working on tTG blockers that would stop tissue transglutaminase so that it does not "attack" gliadin. There are tTG blockers now that have been shown, experimentally, to block inflammation in animal models.

However, tTG is an enzyme that is present in every tissue of the body and is crucial for many bodily functions. Any tTG blocker would have to work only in the intestine and then be rapidly inactivated. Of interest, mice have been developed that are genetically devoid of tTG (tTG knockout mice). These mice have a normal appearance—raising the possibility that we could, in fact, live without tTG.

One such drug, TG2ZED-1337, is in clinical studies in Europe with results to be presented in the very near future.

Designer Drugs

Sitting in the Groove

Moving down the sequence of events, the next targets for drug action are the molecules that are the genetic markers for the disease, HLA-DQ2 and HLA-DQ8. HLA-DQ2 and HLA-DQ8 molecules sit on the surface of specific cells (antigen-presenting cells, APC) looking for foreign invaders. They are the site of interaction with the primed gliadin fragment that has been acted upon by tissue transglutaminase. The primed gliadin initiates the immune response by sitting in the pocket or groove on the surface of the HLA-DQ2 or HLA-DQ8 molecule. (See Figure 10, page 73.)

Drugs are being researched that could sit in that groove and block the deamidated gliadin from interacting with HLA-DQ2 and HLA-DQ8, thereby stopping the inflammatory reaction that causes the flattening of the villi. The role of this class of drug in celiac disease has yet to be determined.

Cytokine Blocker

Cytokines are protein messengers found in the body. They play an integral role in inflammation. In celiac disease, they act as important messengers as well as instigators of the inflammatory response. That is, they set off and continue the inflammatory reaction in the small intestine.

Cytokines are released from inflammatory cells and do the damage that results in villous atrophy. A number of cytokines are at work in the intestine, including interleukin 15 (IL-15).

Blocking the Cytokine IL-15

Lymphocytes are one of the main types of immune cells found in the body and are important in active celiac disease. IL-15 revs up the intraepithelial lymphocytes that sit within the cells lining the small intestine. They are the basis of refractory celiac disease type 2, in which the intraepithelial lymphocytes behave in a premalignant way. An antibody to IL-15 has been developed by Amgen for rheumatoid arthritis and shown to be safe and beneficial in patients with active celiac disease and refractory celiac disease type 2. Other companies are developing antibodies to block other cytokines.

Unfortunately, blocking any of the cytokines may also block their good work, and using a cytokine blocker may increase the chances of getting a severe infection that the cytokines protect against.

Again, there are already examples of cytokine blockers being used in medicine, especially inflammatory bowel diseases such as ulcerative colitis and Crohn's disease.

Nanoparticles

Nanoparticles are microscopically small particles that are being used in medicine to deliver drugs and substances to specific cells. As therapeutic delivery systems, nanoparticles allow targeted delivery and controlled release. They are being studied as a means to teach the body to tolerate gluten, similar to a vaccine.

Developed at Northwestern Medicine and now by Takeda Pharmaceutical Company, TAK-101 is a biodegradable nanoparticle containing gluten that aims to teach the immune system that the antigen is safe and to induce tolerance to gluten. The nanoparticle has been described as a "Trojan horse" hiding the gluten allergen in a friendly shell in order to convince the immune system not to attack it. It is administered intravenously and patients in a Phase II clinical trial were then fed gluten for two weeks. The drug was generally safe and well tolerated and more clinical trials are being developed.

At this point in the development of nanoparticle therapy, the potential side effects and toxicities are not well known.

"First, Do No Harm"

As our knowledge of the molecular and biological workings of the gluten molecule on the intestinal wall progresses, so will potential therapies. We need to be optimistic but realistic. Many of the therapies we have described are still theoretical.

It is also possible that people will be able to take more than one medication. Some of the therapies being developed may be complementary and have a more complete effect when used together. **Combination therapy may, in fact, be the treatment future for celiac disease.**

Another issue is cost—whether insurance carriers will pay for these therapies, which will not be cheap.

Drug Trials

The development of drugs is an expensive and lengthy process. Studies show that it costs more than a billion dollars and takes at least ten years to bring a drug to market.

In order to get on the market, the FDA mandates that a medicine needs to make people feel better—that is, reduce symptoms—and cause no harm. Importantly, these benefits need to be demonstrated in rigorous studies. The studies are double-blinded (neither the patient nor the investigator knows who gets the drug) and placebo-controlled (some participants get the drug; others get a placebo). And the studies are overseen by the FDA. There also have to be predetermined endpoints—such as a reduction in symptoms and healing of the biopsy. The FDA also mandates that companies developing therapies for celiac disease prepare studies that include children.

Studies are conducted through several phases:

- Phase I determines that the drug is safe and helps to determine a dosage.
- Phase II determines that the drug is effective in patients, works better than placebo in eliminating symptoms, and protects from damage.
- Phase III expands the number of subjects being tested and assesses effectiveness and safety.

Conducting drug trials in people with celiac disease is very difficult, since being in a study alters behavior. Once enrolled, people are reminded every day that they have celiac disease and need to monitor their adherence to a gluten-free diet. Because this often makes them more adherent than before, it is difficult to determine the difference between the drug and the placebo in stopping symptoms.

Most important, we must ensure that any drug therapy is (1) safe and (2) effective, because the current therapy—a gluten-free diet—is both.

The Future—Prevention of Celiac Disease

While a cure is important and drug therapy necessary, we need to determine why celiac disease is increasing so rapidly and how to prevent the disease in future generations. Prevention is the best therapy of all.

28

Myths and Unexplored Areas

Actual evidence I have none . . .

—R. Arkell, All the Rumours, *1916*

For all of the scientific information about celiac disease that is now available, the number of myths and anecdotal information still circulating is remarkable. Some are passed on by patients or websites and relate to food. Others are dated beliefs held within the medical community.

I was diagnosed the first time when I was three. My younger sister (who was one and a half) and I became extremely ill around the same time. We had conflicting symptoms, which threw the doctor off for a while. Although we both had white bowel movements, I was very puffy, sort of overweight, with a hollow neck and sunken cheeks. My sister looked malnourished—very skinny arms and legs with a huge protruding stomach, and an unnamed rash. She was very lethargic. Eventually, a doctor in Boston thought it might be something called "tropical sprue." He told my mother: "You have to be their doctor, take them off of gluten, write down everything they eat, and just hope."

We ate rice and potatoes, lots of vegetables . . . we stayed away from dairy. We did this until we were thirteen. Initially, we were given shots of gamma globulin, and then B_{12} shots on a regular basis. We were told we would outgrow it, and, eventually, we both became asymptomatic—so we came off the diet.

*My health slowly declined over the eighteen years between di-
agnoses. In 1982, I had a series of blood tests and was told I had
secondary malnutrition; I was anemic; I had a lot of intestinal problems. I told the doctor I had celiac disease as a child and asked if it
could be back. He said: "No, you outgrew that." He prescribed vitamins, but I didn't feel better. I gave up trying to solve the problem
and figured this was the way life was going to be.*

*By 1986, I was diagnosed with IBS (irritable bowel syndrome)
and spastic colon. My menstrual cycle was very out of whack. I
didn't want to go on any sort of hormones; I just dealt with it. And
I had horrible depression—that was probably the worst part.*

*By 1989, I dropped down to ninety-two pounds (I'm 5'5").
Nothing stayed in my body. That's when I was finally rediagnosed
with celiac disease. I had been so sick for so long, the diagnosis
was a relief. I went back to the way I ate as a child. I did a lot of juic-
ing those first few months while my intestines healed.*

*There's a generation out there who think, or were told, they out-
grew it. They're adults now, and they don't want to hear about celiac
disease. I lost eighteen years of proper care—which has definitely
affected my life. If I had known that you never outgrow it, I never
would have gone off the diet.* (Ceil, 43)

Myths Surrounding Celiac Disease

Myth #1: You Can Outgrow Celiac Disease.

Celiac disease is a hereditary, autoimmune disease that may become
asymptomatic after a period of time on a gluten-free diet. It does *not*
mean you have outgrown it, just that it has become silent—and may re-
surface in the form of ancillary autoimmune conditions, malignancies,
infertility, or other manifestations. There are individuals who had celiac
disease as a child and were told that they had "outgrown it." We see them
at the Center when they develop cancer of the small intestine in their fifties due to a lifelong active celiac disease that was asymptomatic. The diagnosis of celiac disease requires a *lifelong* adherence to a gluten-free
diet to avoid complications.

Myth #2: A Little Bit of Gluten Every Now and Then Will Not Hurt.

I think there's a lot of distrust on the part of some of the adults. They were the IBS (irritable bowel syndrome) type of people, who always had a bad stomach, a lot of diarrhea. They got to their forties and fifties with these symptoms and finally got this diagnosis of celiac disease. They don't stay on the diet and don't really believe that they have it (celiac disease). I find all these adults are really lax, and if they feel sick after eating a bagel, they don't care. They think they've been misdiagnosed—that it's bull. There's huge denial of it. I don't think they understand the ramifications of celiac disease. (Sue, 41)

Researchers have shown that ingesting 100 milligrams of gluten a day will cause continued damage to the villi of the intestine. While the exact amount of gluten that can be ingested daily without causing intestinal damage has not been scientifically proved, a recent study from Finland calculates it to be about 30 milligrams. Put differently, this is substantially *less* than a teaspoon of birthday cake.

Myth #3: You Do Not Need a Biopsy.

Two of my sisters and I were diagnosed with celiac disease by the same pediatrician in Brooklyn. We were all banana babies. My other siblings went to a different pediatrician and were told they never had it. Yet when I was recently tested—I was having stomachaches and problems—and biopsied, I was told I never had celiac disease. I wish we were all evaluated properly as children. It would have prevented a lot of stress and expense on the part of my parents. And guilt! (Paul, 35)

A biopsy remains the gold standard for diagnosis. Other disease processes can cause the same symptoms, and eliminating gluten from the diet often improves them as well. A trial gluten-free diet should be avoided.

Intestinal biopsy has been in use since the 1950s. It is now easy and safe to do one, even on small children. Physicians need to be *very* certain of the diagnosis to place anyone on a gluten-free diet for life. Ask for a biopsy!

Myth #4: Vinegar Contains Gluten.

Any vinegar that is distilled is gluten-free. Malt vinegar is not distilled and contains gluten. It is important to read labels to see what other ingredients may be in a product that contains vinegar. But the distilled vinegar itself is not an offending ingredient.

Myth #5: Distilled Alcohol Contains Gluten.

The distilling process eliminates the gliadin fragment from spirits made from wheat, rye, and barley (e.g., bourbon, vodka, scotch). If spirits contain flavoring that is added in after the alcohol is distilled, it is not necessarily safe. Beer is brewed, not distilled, and is therefore not safe. (There are, however, gluten-free beers on the market.)

Myth #6: Gluten Is Absorbed Through the Skin.

Gluten needs to react with intestinal immune cells to initiate the inflammatory process. You would have to drink a shampoo or skin lotion to cause the intestinal damage seen in celiac disease.

Similarly, dermatitis herpetiformis, the skin manifestation of celiac disease, is not triggered by topical applications of creams and lotions containing gluten. These potions may aggravate an existing skin condition—or cause an allergic reaction, which is a different disease process—but they cannot cause dermatitis herpetiformis. If specific products irritate or inflame your skin, you should stop using them. But do not blame them for causing celiac disease or dermatitis herpetiformis.

Myth #7: You Can Get Celiac Disease Through a Blood Transfusion.

There is an erroneous belief that the antibodies that are found in the blood can cause celiac disease and, therefore, can be passed along through a blood transfusion. The antibodies to gluten made by people with celiac disease are bystanders and not part of the damaging process. Even if the antibodies were passed on to someone during a transfusion, they can neither cause damage nor bestow protection from celiac disease.

Myth #8: I Saw It on the Internet.

Scientific information is the only form of information that a patient should rely upon. It is important to separate medically driven and properly researched information from opinion. Anecdotes from other patients and/or postings that begin "I read somewhere that . . ." should be suspect until proved otherwise. Patients must make up their own minds about a number of issues raised in this book. But these decisions should be based upon science, not on opinions posted by someone who got violently ill after ingesting a supposedly gluten-free product.

Unexplored Areas

While research is in the works on a number of fronts, there are many intriguing questions that remain to be examined. These include, but are not limited to, the following:

What Are the Mechanisms/Causes of Celiac Disease?

Researchers have probed into the lining of the small intestine, as well as the layers of the skin, and uncovered a great deal of information about the causes and development of celiac disease and dermatitis herpetiformis. A great deal more remains to be uncovered, including:

- What accounts for the incredibly varied manifestations of the disease?
- What are all the genes responsible for celiac disease, and do the different genes account for the varied manifestations?
- How does breast-feeding prevent or modify the clinical presentation of celiac disease?

What Is the Role of Serologic Testing (Blood Tests) and How Can It Be Standardized?

The standardization of tests—and test kits—is important so that interpretation can be compared and interlaboratory variation minimized. This will also eliminate some of the inconclusive results that leave patients and doctors unsure of both diagnosis and treatment.

Perhaps better tests can be developed that would be sufficient to diagnose celiac disease without a biopsy.

How Much Gluten Is Too Much?

Still unresolved, this is a pivotal issue for every patient. Will cross contamination prevent healing, and if not, what is the acceptable level of gluten that can safely be ingested? More research is necessary.

What Are the Genetic Links?

There are probably multiple genes that play a role in celiac disease in addition to the HLA-DQ2 and HLA-DQ8 genes. Uncovering these other genes may impact research into a possible cure or "blocker" for the disease.

If Celiac Disease Is So Common, Why Did Those Genes Get Encouraged?

It is postulated that celiac disease somehow conveyed a survival advantage. A study of refugee populations in northern Africa suggested that the damaged intestine offered less surface area for bacterial infections to bind onto and cause diarrhea. Therefore, fewer children died from chronic diarrhea commonly found in developing countries. Celiac disease was protective in that respect.

Patients with active celiac disease tend to have low cholesterol levels because they are not properly absorbing cholesterol in the intestine. Does this infer less cardiovascular disease? And did this somehow convey a survival advantage? Arguing against this theory is the fact that, until the twentieth century, most people died of infections and/or trauma well before they were old enough to develop cardiovascular disease, today's major killer.

What Are the Long-Term Effects of Undiagnosed Celiac Disease?

While a lowered cholesterol level is a positive effect, this must be weighed against the increased potential to develop a chronic disease such as osteoporosis, diabetes, and some malignancies.

What Is the Prevalence and Clinical Impact of Celiac Disease in Non-European Populations?

Celiac disease was once considered to be a condition that mainly affected people of European descent. Recent studies on the international face of the disease show that to be inaccurate. Cases of celiac disease have been reported in children from Eastern Europe; North, West, and East Africa; southern and central Asia; and the Middle East. Celiac disease is truly a worldwide disease.

The potential for celiac disease to become a major health issue in developing countries is highlighted by the report of the high rate of celiac disease in a population of refugee children in North Africa. This raises important health issues because the major grain supplied to refugee populations is wheat that is produced in excess by developed countries.

There are no studies that have specifically screened African American, Hispanic, or Native American populations in the United States. A recent study from Canada described celiac disease among Asian Canadians with origins from northern India, Japan, and China.

Celiac disease is seen in many patients from developing countries, both in their native lands and as immigrants in developed countries. This has important implications for medical practitioners throughout the world.

What Is the Effect of a Gluten-Free Diet on Other Conditions, and the Brain?

Gluten has been targeted and researched as a possible agent or trigger in a wide variety of conditions, both physical and psychological. While most of the connections have not been well established, it is very possible that gluten/gliadin may play a role in many diseases. Research into the mind/body role of inflammation and the gluten connection will ultimately impact the patient population with celiac disease.

Should Everyone Be Diagnosed and Treated?

Celiac disease fulfills the World Health Organization (WHO) criteria for screening for a disease:

1. It is a condition that is an important health problem whose development is understood.
2. It can be safely and accurately diagnosed.
3. There is an effective treatment for it.
4. There is a benefit to and cost-effective reason for treatment.

Nevertheless, screening populations means that you are testing people who may feel healthy and then telling them that they have a disease.

A study from Finland showed an increased quality of life for people diagnosed through screening. This suggests that even though people may not think they are ill and seek health care, they are better off being diagnosed with celiac disease if they do have it. However, not all studies agree on this point—many people show no improvement because they felt well to begin with—and a British study demonstrated that some people diagnosed by screening regretted being diagnosed.

On one hand, early diagnosis improves the long-term health of people with celiac disease and prevents further complications and progression.

Conversely, there will be a longer period of treatment, higher costs involved in the management of the disease, and potentially false-positive and false-negative diagnoses. There is also an ethical dilemma: Do parents who subject their children to testing have the right *not* to treat their apparently healthy child with a restrictive diet and altered lifestyle?

Can researchers identify the people who are not going to do well—those who will develop lymphomas and multiple autoimmune conditions—and distinguish them from those who will not develop the more severe consequences of celiac disease? Is it genes or another factor(s) that turns celiac disease into a major medical situation versus a discomforting chronic condition with a few ancillary problems? Until it is possible to identify these patients, we advise all those diagnosed—with or without symptoms—to follow a strict gluten-free diet.

What Is the Future for Home Test Kits?

Home test kits (see Chapter 4) for IgA tissue transglutaminase (tTG) antibodies and genetic markers are being marketed directly to the consumer. Ideally, they will increase the diagnosis of celiac disease. These kits, which put test results in the hands of the patient, raise several issues that need to be addressed:

- What will patients do with the information?
- Will they seek professional help before self-treating?
- Will they receive adequate counseling from health care professionals regarding the significance of the results? For example, how will false positives and false negatives be explained and handled?

Medical home test kits have been available for many years, the home pregnancy test being a prime example. But women who get a positive result on a pregnancy test routinely make their next stop a visit to the obstetrician/gynecologist. We hope that a gastroenterologist or internist will be consulted by anyone using home tests for celiac disease.

Why Isn't Celiac Disease More Common?

With few exceptions, we all eat wheat in one form or another. The important HLA genes that predispose people to celiac disease occur in 30 to 40 percent of the Western population. The protective mucosal barrier of the small intestine is regularly disrupted by infections, medications, smoking, and alcohol, potentially letting gliadin in. All of this equals a perfect storm for the creation of celiac disease, yet celiac disease only occurs in 1 percent of the population.

Studies of stored blood samples from at-risk children followed from birth have shown that some individuals may go through periods of gluten autoimmunity or celiac disease that does not persist. This indicates that there is a give-and-take in the destructive and protective immune reactions in any individual and that in some, gluten intolerance may be temporary.

An intriguing area for future study will be determining the protective mechanisms that enable a large percentage of wheat-consuming people, with a genetic predisposition and an occasionally "leaky gut," to avoid celiac disease.

What Will the Future Involve?

As more people are diagnosed we will see:

- A greater awareness of the disease
- A greater variety of and ease in obtaining gluten-free food
- An increased ability to enjoy a more normal, less stressful life
- A better idea among the medical community of the prognosis and treatment of the disease

As knowledge of celiac disease grows, the feelings of isolation felt by many people should diminish. Life will become easier as more people are diagnosed, restaurants become more accommodating, gluten-free products are more widely available (and less expensive), and scientific and dietary information is more uniform.

The gluten-free diet offers health to many people who have suffered for years before being diagnosed. So, while some people continue to wait for a cure, others feel they already have one.

A Guide to Ingredients

By Ann Whelan and Amy Ratner
Editors, *Gluten-Free Living*

The information below is based on extensive product research through contact with both food scientists and processors. Some of the ingredients are safe (gluten-free), some are unsafe (not gluten-free), and a few are questionable. This information will help you read a food label.

Caramel color
Although FDA regulations permit the use of malt syrup to make caramel color, processors in the United States almost always use corn because it makes a better product. It is gluten-free.

Citric acid
This ingredient is gluten-free. It is usually made from corn, beet sugar, or molasses. Even when made from wheat, citric acid is so highly processed and purified that no gluten protein would remain.

Dextrin
Dextrin made from corn, potato, arrowroot, rice, or tapioca is gluten-free. It can be made from wheat, though this is rare, and would not be gluten-free. If dextrin is made from wheat, "wheat" will appear on the label.

Dextrose
An ingredient made from starch, including rice, corn, or wheat. It is a highly processed ingredient that is gluten-free no matter which starch is used.

Flavors (artificial and natural)

Flavors are rarely made from gluten-containing grains, according to the Flavor and Extract Manufacturers Association. If wheat is used to make a flavor, "wheat" must appear on the label. Some flavoring is made with ethanol that comes from wheat. In that case, the flavor would still be gluten-free because ethanol is distilled, which removes the gluten protein.

Glucose syrup

A gluten-free sweetener made most frequently from corn, but also from tapioca, potato, sorghum, or wheat starch. It is such a highly processed and purified ingredient that the source of the starch does not matter. Even if you see glucose syrup derived from wheat on a label, it is still gluten-free.

Guar gum

A gluten-free thickening ingredient made from the guar bean. It is used in gluten-free baking to help provide the stretch that normally comes from gluten. It can work like a laxative if consumed in large quantities.

Herbs

All plain herbs are gluten-free.

Hydrolyzed vegetable protein (HVP) and hydrolyzed plant protein (HPP)

The source of the protein should always be listed on the label of a food that contains HVP or HPP. If it is "hydrolyzed soy protein," it is gluten-free. If it is "hydrolyzed wheat protein," it is not gluten-free.

Lecithin

Used to thicken food, lecithin is usually made from soy and is gluten-free.

Malt

Although it can be made from corn, malt flavoring is usually made from barley and is not gluten-free. Labels do not have to specify the source of malt flavoring but some companies voluntarily note which grain is used. Malt extract, malt flavoring, malt syrup, and malt flour are also made from barley. None of these ingredients are safe. (See Vinegar, page 298.)

Maltodextrin

Maltodextrin is gluten-free. It can be made from a variety of starches, including corn, potato, rice, or wheat. However, the source does not matter because maltodextrin is such a highly processed ingredient that the protein is removed, rendering it gluten-free. If wheat is used, "wheat" will appear on the label. Even in this case, the maltodextrin would be gluten-free.

Modified food starch

An ingredient made from a variety of starches. Modified food starch is gluten-free unless it is made from wheat. If it is made from wheat, "wheat" will appear on the label. Many companies are listing all sources of modified food starch voluntarily.

Mono- and diglycerides

Mono- and diglycerides are fats and are gluten-free.

MSG

Monosodium glutamate is a flavoring made through the fermentation of corn, sugar, beets, or sugarcane. It is gluten-free.

Oat gum

Oat gum is rarely used as an ingredient. It is made from the carbohydrate portion of oats. Since gluten is a protein, oat gum would be gluten-free.

Seasonings

Seasonings (and seasoning mixes) can contain a wide variety of ingredients. Some are not gluten-free because they contain wheat flour or wheat starch, which will be noted on the label. Others contain only spices, herbs, and gluten-free ingredients and are gluten-free.

Seitan

An ingredient found in vegetarian food that is made from wheat gluten.

Soy sauce

Most brands of soy sauce contain wheat, which will be listed on the label. Some brands contain only soybeans and are gluten-free.

Spices

Pure spices are gluten-free. Some contain silicon dioxide, which is gluten-free and used to keep the spice free-flowing.

Starch

On food labels, "starch" always means cornstarch and is gluten-free.

Vanilla

A gluten-free flavoring made from distilled alcohol and flavor extracted from the vanilla seed (pure extract) or from artificial vanilla flavoring (artificial extract). Distillation removes the gluten protein from the alcohol.

Vinegar

Distilled vinegar is gluten-free and has always been gluten-free. The only vinegar to avoid is malt vinegar, which is made from barley and is not distilled. There is no evidence that suggests vinegar might be dangerous for those who follow the gluten-free diet.

Whey

The liquid part of milk that separates from solids when cheese is made. It is used as an additive in many processed foods and is gluten-free.

Yeast

All brand-name packaged yeasts sold in the United States are gluten-free. Autolyzed yeast in a food product is generally considered gluten-free. Brewer's yeast, when it is a by-product of beer, is not considered gluten-free. However, brewer's yeast nutritional supplements can be made from either brewer's yeast or sugar. If made from sugar, they are gluten-free.

Explanation of Grains

Most people are not familiar with the wide variety of grains now commonly available. Many are staples of other cuisines and easily purchased in ethnic or health food stores.

Do not be intimidated by unusual names and new flavors. They are just as easy to cook and just as delicious as old standbys. Many of the grains are also packed with nutrients and a desirable alternative to rice, corn, and potatoes in the gluten-free diet.

These nutritious grains should be included regularly for young children who are growing up gluten-free. They can add needed nutrients and, if introduced early with other new foods, avoid the "strangeness" of flavor many adults confront.

Use grains as hot cereal, side dishes, in soups and stews, as flour for pancakes and baked products, and so forth. Many are also commonly found as cold cereal.

Amaranth. Once a sacred food of the Aztecs, amaranth has a cornlike aroma and woodsy flavor. It is well suited to porridge-type dishes or ground into flour for bread. It is high in protein, dietary fiber, iron, magnesium, zinc, calcium, and B vitamins.

Buckwheat. The grain has a nutty flavor and makes a delicious hot cereal or side dish. It can be added to salads, stuffings, soups, stews, and casseroles, and its small, nutty kernels are an interesting replacement for barley. Buckwheat is called "kasha" when the seeds have been roasted; grits are coarsely ground buckwheat seeds or groats.

It is also available in flour form—which is sometimes mixed with wheat flour—for baking, pancakes, and thickeners. Read labels carefully. Soba noodles are a blend of buckwheat and wheat flour. Buckwheat is gluten-free, but the flour may be cross contaminated or mixed; thus, you should consult the manufacturers before selecting their product. There are mills* that specialize in this grain.

It is high in high-quality protein, magnesium, B_6, dietary fiber, iron, niacin, thiamin, and zinc.

Millet. Dry and airy when cooked with a little water, millet is also moist and dense when cooked with extra water. Bland in flavor, millet readily takes on the flavors of foods cooked with it. This grain is a good hot cereal (with honey or seasoning) or side dish, and it can be used as flour in baking. It is high in protein and fiber.

Quinoa. A native South American grain with a soft, crunchy texture, quinoa boasts the highest nutritional profile of all grains. It is often called a "super grain." This grain can be mixed with onions, nuts, or vegetables as a delicious side dish. It contains more high-quality protein than other grains and cereals and is also high in iron, magnesium, B vitamins, and calcium.

Teff. Teff can be used as a hot cereal or side dish, and it is good in casseroles, or cold as a salad. There are teff pastas available, and it is also available as flour, which can be used to thicken sauces. It is high in protein, calcium, iron, and B vitamins.

Wild rice. The taste, aroma, size, and color of wild rice—typically black, brown, or red—depend on whether it is wild or cultivated, where it is harvested, and how it is processed. It adds crunch, color, and a nutty flavor to rice dishes. Mixed with white rice, a small amount of wild rice—which can be expensive—goes a long way. It makes an excellent addition to both hot and cold side dishes. It has dietary fiber, protein, potassium, and zinc.

---

* In the United States, the following mills deal with buckwheat: Bouchard Family Farms (800-239-3237), Birkett Mills (315-536-3311), New Hope Mills (315-252-2676), Arrowhead Mills (800-434-4246). Most claim that their buckwheat is gluten-free; some mill *only* buckwheat.

APPENDIX C

Books and Articles of Interest

BOOKS

There are many excellent cookbooks and advice books that deal with various aspects of the gluten-free diet. This short list is only a suggested sampling of medical, dietary, and/or lifestyle books that provide a good base of knowledge upon which to build.

Case S. *Gluten-Free: The Definitive Resource Guide* (Fifth Edition). Regina, Saskatchewan: Case Nutrition Consulting; 2016.

Diamond JM. *Guns, Germs, and Steel: The Fates of Human Societies.* New York: W. W. Norton & Company; 1997.

Groopman J. *How Doctors Think.* New York: Mariner Books; 2008.

Mahan LK, Raymond JL, eds. *Krause's Food and the Nutrition Care Process.* 14th ed. Philadelphia, PA: W. B. Saunders Company; 2017.

Shomon MJ. *Living Well with Autoimmune Disease.* New York: Harper Resource; 2001.

Vander AJ, Sherman JH, Luciano DS. *Human Physiology: The Mechanisms of Body Function.* 7th ed. New York: McGraw-Hill; 1998.

PEER REVIEW PUBLICATIONS

Most of Dr. Green's articles are available through the website of the Celiac Disease Center at Columbia: www.celiacdiseasecenter.columbia.edu.

All of the following publications may not be readily accessible. The abstract, or summary, of the article is available on: www.pubmed.gov.

REVIEWS ON CELIAC DISEASE

Aziz I, Hadjivassiliou M, Sanders DS. The spectrum of non-coeliac gluten sensitivity. *Nat Rev Gastroenterol Hepatol.* 2015 Sep;12(9):516–26.

Clappison E, Hadjivassiliou M, Zis P. Psychiatric manifestations of coeliac disease: a systematic review and meta-analysis. *Nutrients.* 2020 Jan 4; 12(1).

Green PHR, Guandalini S. When is celiac disease celiac disease? *Gastroenterology.* 2019 Aug;157(2):293–94.

Iversen R, Sollid LM. Autoimmunity provoked by foreign antigens. *Science.* 2020 Apr 10;368(6487):132–33.

Lebwohl B, Sanders DS, Green PHR. Coeliac disease. *Lancet.* 2018 Jan 6;391(10115):70–81.

Zylberberg HM, Lebwohl B, Green PHR. Celiac disease—musculoskeletal manifestations and mechanisms in children to adults. *Curr Osteoporos Rep.* 2018 Dec;16(6):754–62.

CURRENT PAPERS OF NOTE

Abadie V, Kim SM, Lejeune T, Palanski BA, Ernest JD, Tastet O, Voisine J, Discepolo V, Marietta EV, Hawash MBF, Ciszewski C, Bouziat R, Panigrahi K, Horwath I, Zurenski MA, Lawrence I, Dumaine A, Yotova V, Grenier JC, Murray JA, Khosla C, Barreiro LB, Jabri B. IL-15, gluten and HLA-DQ8 drive tissue destruction in coeliac disease. *Nature.* 2020 Feb;578(7796):600–604.

Altenbach SB, Chang HC, Rowe MH, Yu XB, Simon-Buss A, Seabourn BW, Green PH, Alaedini A. Reducing the immunogenic potential of wheat flour: silencing of alpha gliadin genes in a U.S. wheat cultivar. *Front Plant Sci.* 2020 Feb 25;11:20.

Al-Toma A, Volta U, Auricchio R, Castillejo G, Sanders DS, Cellier C, Mulder CJ, Lundin KEA. European Society for the Study of Coeliac Disease (ESsCD) guideline for coeliac disease and other gluten-related disorders. *United European Gastroenterol J.* 2019 Jun;7(5):583–613. doi: 10.1177/2050640619844125. Epub 2019 Apr 13. Review.

Andrén Aronsson C, Lee HS, Hård Af Segerstad EM, Uusitalo U, Yang J, Koletzko S, Liu E, Kurppa K, Bingley PJ, Toppari J, Ziegler AG, She JX, Hagopian WA, Rewers M, Akolkar B, Krischer JP, Virtanen SM, Norris JM, Agardh D; TEDDY Study Group. Association of gluten intake during the first 5 years of life with incidence of celiac disease autoimmunity and celiac disease among children at increased risk. *JAMA.* 2019 Aug 13;322(6):514–23.

Bouziat R, Hinterleitner R, Brown JJ, Stencel-Baerenwald JE, Ikizler M, Mayassi T, Meisel M, Kim SM, Discepolo V, Pruijssers AJ, Ernest JD, Iskarpatyoti JA, Costes LM, Lawrence I, Palanski BA, Varma M, Zurenski MA, Khomandiak S, McAllister N, Aravamudhan P, Boehme KW, Hu F, Samsom JN, Reinecker HC, Kupfer SS, Guandalini S, Semrad CE, Abadie V, Khosla C, Barreiro LB, Xavier RJ, Ng A, Dermody TS, Jabri B. Reovirus infection triggers inflammatory responses to dietary antigens and development of celiac disease. *Science.* 2017 Apr 7; 356(6333):44–50.

Cadenhead JW, Wolf RL, Lebwohl B, Lee AR, Zybert P, Reilly NR, Schebendach J, Satherley R, Green PHR. Diminished quality of life among adolescents with coeliac disease using maladaptive eating behaviours to manage a gluten-free diet: a cross-sectional, mixed-methods study. *J Hum Nutr Diet.* 2019 Jun;32(3):311–20. doi: 10.1111/jhn.12638. Epub 2019 Mar.

Cellier C, Bouma G, van Gils T, Khater S, Malamut G, Crespo L, Collin P, Green PHR, Crowe SE, Tsuji W, Butz E, Cerf-Bensussan N, Macintyre E, Parnes JR, Leon F, Hermine O, Mulder CJ; RCD-II Study Group Investigators. Safety and efficacy of AMG 714 in patients with type 2 refractory coeliac disease: a phase 2a, randomised, double-blind, placebo-controlled, parallel-group study. *Lancet Gastroenterol Hepatol.* 2019 Sep 4. pii: S2468-1253(19)30265-1. doi: 1016/S2468-1253(19)30265-1.

Croall ID, Sanders DS, Hadjivassiliou M, Hoggard N. Cognitive deficit and white matter changes in persons with celiac disease: a population-based study. *Gastroenterology.* 2020 Feb 20. pii: S0016-5085(20)30 239-0.

Joelson AM, Geller MG, Zylberberg HM, Green PHR, Lebwohl B. Numbers and features of patients with a diagnosis of celiac disease without duodenal biopsy, based on a national survey. *Clin Gastroenterol Hepatol.* 2018 Sep 10. pii: S1542-3565(18)30967-4. doi: 10.1016/j.cgh.2018.09 .006.

Laszkowska M, Mahadev S, Sundström J, Lebwohl B, Green PHR, Michaelsson K, Ludvigsson JF. Systematic review with meta-analysis: the prevalence of coeliac disease in patients with osteoporosis. *Aliment Pharmacol Ther.* 2018 Jul 8. doi: 10.1111/apt.14911.29984519.

Lebwohl B, Green PHR, Söderling J, Roelstraete B, Ludvigsson JF. Association between celiac disease and mortality risk in a Swedish population. *JAMA*. 2020 Apr 7;323(13):1277–85.

Lebwohl B, Nobel YR, Green PHR, Blaser MJ, Ludvigsson JF. Risk of Clostridium difficile infection in patients with celiac disease: a population-based study. *Am J Gastroenterol*. 2017 Dec;112(12):1878–84.

Lebwohl B, Roy A, Alaedini A, Green PHR, Ludvigsson JF. Risk of headache-related healthcare visits in patients with celiac disease: a population-based observational study. *Headache*. 2016 May;56(5): 849–58.

Lee AR, Wolf RL, Lebwohl B, Ciaccio EJ, Green PHR. Persistent economic burden of the gluten free diet. *Nutrients*. 2019 Feb 14;11(2). doi: 10.3390/nu11020399.

Lerner BA, Phan Vo LT, Yates S, Rundle AG, Green PHR, Lebwohl B. Detection of gluten in gluten-free labeled restaurant food: analysis of crowd-sourced data. *Am J Gastroenterol*. 2019 Mar 26.

Liu E, Dong F, Barón AE, Taki I, Norris JM, Frohnert BI, Hoffenberg EJ, Rewers M. High incidence of celiac disease in a long-term study of adolescents with susceptibility genotypes. *Gastroenterology*. 2017 May; 152(6):1329–36.

Ludvigsson JF, Lebwohl B, Chen Q, Bröms G, Wolf RL, Green PHR, Emilsson L. Anxiety after coeliac disease diagnosis predicts mucosal healing: a population-based study. *Aliment Pharmacol Ther*. 2018 Nov; 48(10):1091–98. doi: 10.1111/apt.14991.

Mahadev S, Laszkowska M, Sundström J, Björkholm M, Lebwohl B, Green PHR, Ludvigsson JF. Prevalence of celiac disease in patients with iron deficiency anemia: a systematic review with meta-analysis. *Gastroenterology*. 2018 Aug;155(2):374–382.e1. doi: 10.1053/j.gastro.2018.04.016.

Myléus A, Reilly NR, Green PHR. Rate, risk factors, and outcomes of nonadherence in pediatric patients with celiac disease: a systematic review. *Clin Gastroenterol Hepatol*. 2019 Jun 4. pii: S1542-3565(19)30597-X. doi: 10.1016/j.cgh.2019.05.046.

Pinto-Sánchez MI, Causada-Calo N, Bercik P, Ford AC, Murray JA, Armstrong D, Semrad C, Kupfer SS, Alaedini A, Moayyedi P, Leffler DA, Verdú EF, Green P. Safety of adding oats to a gluten-free diet for patients with celiac disease: systematic review and meta-analysis of clinical and observational studies. *Gastroenterology*. 2017 Aug;153(2): 395–409.

Reilly NR, Hammer ML, Ludvigsson JF, Green PH. Frequency and predictors of successful transition of care for young adults with childhood celiac disease. *J Pediatr Gastroenterol Nutr.* 2020 Feb;70(2):190–94.

Roy A, Laszkowska M, Sundström J, Lebwohl B, Green PH, Kämpe O, Ludvigsson JF. Prevalence of celiac disease in patients with autoimmune thyroid disease: a meta-analysis. *Thyroid.* 2016 Jul;26(7):880–90.

Roy A, Minaya M, Monegro M, Fleming J, Wong RK, Lewis S, Lebwohl B, Green PH. Partner burden: a common entity in celiac disease. *Dig Dis Sci.* 2016 Dec;61(12):3451–59. Epub 2016.

Walker MD, Williams J, Lewis SK, Bai JC, Lebwohl B, Green PH. Measurement of forearm bone density by dual energy X-ray absorptiometry increases the prevalence of osteoporosis in men with celiac disease. *Clin Gastroenterol Hepatol.* 2019 Apr 10. doi: 10.1016/j.cgh.2019.03.049. Epub ahead of print.

Wolf RL, Green PHR, Lee AR, Reilly NR, Zybert P, Lebwohl B. Benefits from and barriers to portable detection of gluten, based on a randomized pilot trial of patients with celiac disease. *Clin Gastroenterol Hepatol.* 2019 Mar 15. doi: 10.1016/j.cgh.2019.03.011. Epub ahead of print.

Zylberberg HM, Ludvigsson JF, Green PHR, Lebwohl B. Psychotropic medication use among patients with celiac disease. *BMC Psychiatry.* 2018 Mar 27;18(1):76.

Resources

MANUFACTURERS OF GLUTEN-FREE PRODUCTS

The past few years have seen an enormous increase in the variety and availability of gluten-free foods. There are now gluten-free breads, crackers, pizzas, pastas, cookies, and cakes to please almost every palate. While many of these are more expensive than their wheat-based counterparts, the product mix is now diverse and more readily available in retail stores (both supermarkets and health food stores) as well as online.

The following is a partial list of companies and markets that offer a selection of gluten-free foods. Not all of the companies make and/or sell gluten-free foods exclusively. And many regularly expand their product lines. Inclusion in this list is neither an endorsement nor a guarantee of the products. An asterisk (*) by the company signifies that the products mentioned are processed in a dedicated facility and/or made on dedicated equipment.

Absolutely Gluten Free
www.absolutelygf.com
Gluten-free crackers, pizza, flatbreads, and snacks.

Amy's Kitchen, Inc.
www.amys.com
Frozen and prepared meals and products (available in most retail stores).

Annie's
www.annies.com
A line of gluten-free mac and cheese, fruit snacks, granola bars, and cookies.

Arrowhead Mills

www.arrowheadmills.com

Flours, mixes, and packaged dried products.

* Authentic Foods

www.authenticfoods.com

Baking mixes and supplies, as well as flours. They are a gluten-free specialty producer.

Banza Pasta

www.eatbanza.com

High-protein pasta made from chickpeas.

* Barilla

www.barilla.com/gluten-free-pasta

A gluten-free blend of corn and rice pastas.

Beers

Beer Advocate

www.beeradvocate.com

General information and ratings on beers.

Bard's Beer

www.bardsbeer.com

Epic Brewing Company

http://epicbrewing.com

Estrella Damm

www.estrelladamm.com

Green's Gluten-Free Beers

http://glutenfreebeers.co.uk

Ground Breaker Brewing

www.groundbreakerbrewing.com

Lakefront Brewery

www.lakefrontbrewery.com

New Planet Gluten-Free Beer

www.newplanetbeer.com

Omission Brewing Company
http://omissionbeer.com

Ramapo Valley Brewery
www.rvbrewery.com

Redbridge (Anheuser-Busch)
www.anheuser-busch.com

Sprecher Brewing Co.
www.sprecherbrewery.com

Steadfast Beer Co.
http://steadfastbeer.com

Birkett Mills
www.thebirkettmills.com
Largest manufacturer of buckwheat products.

* Bob's Red Mill
www.bobsredmill.com
Gluten-free products including flours and baking mixes.

* Breads from Anna
www.breadsfromanna.com
Bread mixes made from a variety of wholesome grains.

Canyon Bakehouse
http://canyonglutenfree.com
Bakery products.

* Chebe
www.chebe.com
Mixes and frozen dough that can be made into a number of products.

Country Life (vitamins)
www.countrylifevitamins.com
Certified gluten-free supplement brand.

Cup 4 Cup
www.cup4cup.com
Gluten-free flour blends (allowing for easy one-to-one all-purpose flour
substitution).

* Ener-G Foods, Inc.
www.ener-g.com
Ready-made foods and mixes for diet-restricted individuals. Products are also certified kosher.

* Enjoy Life Foods
http://enjoylifefoods.com
Cookies, bars, and fruit/seed mixes that are free of the top eight allergens.

Freeda Health LLC
www.freedavitamins.com
Gluten-free vitamins.

General Mills
www.generalmills.com
More than six hundred gluten-free products, including cereals, crackers, nutritional bars, dessert mixes, under brand names that include Chex, Betty Crocker, and Bisquick, to name a few.

* The Gluten Free Bakery
www.odbefree.com
Breads and cookies.

The Gluten-Free Mall
www.glutenfreemall.com
Internet "shopping mall" for hundreds of gluten-free products.

Gluten Solutions
www.glutensolutions.com
Another Internet "grocery store" for hundreds of gluten-free products.

Glutino
www.glutino.com
A gluten-free specialty company. Products include baking mixes, cookies, breads, pizza, and more.

Health Valley
www.healthvalley.com
Assortment of "natural" products, some of which are gluten-free.

* Hodgson Mill
www.hodgsonmill.com
Gluten-free products and mixes.

King Arthur Baking
www.kingarthurflour.com
Flours and baking mixes.

* Kinnikinnick Foods, Inc.
www.kinnikinnick.com
A gluten-free specialty company. They produce a variety of products for people with special dietary requirements.

* Lärabar
www.larabar.com
All-natural bars that are a blend of unsweetened fruits, nuts, and spices.

Le Veneziane Pasta
https://molinodiferro.com/
A range of corn pastas from Italy. Available online and in many specialty stores.

Luce's Gluten-Free Artisan Bread Mix
www.lucegfbread.com
Bread and pancake mixes.

* Mary's Gone Crackers
www.marysgonecrackers.com
Organic whole grain gluten-free, wheat-free, and dairy-free crackers, cookies, and snacks.

* Namaste Foods
www.namastefoods.com
Baking and cooking mixes that contain no wheat, gluten, corn, soy, potato, dairy, casein, peanuts, or tree nuts.

* Nana's Cookie Company
www.nanascookiecompany.com
Gluten-free cookies that are also free of corn, soy, dairy, eggs, casein, and wheat.

Nature Made (vitamins)
www.naturemade.com
Gluten-free vitamins.

Nature's Path Foods, Inc.

www.naturespath.com

Organic products made from whole grains. Their gluten-free products are tested, and are available in many retail stores under brand names that include Envirokidz, Nature's Path Foods, and Love Crunch.

Oats (produced in dedicated facilities)

    Bob's Red Mill

    www.bobsredmill.com (note package labels, as some of their products are not gluten-free)

    GF Harvest Oats
    www.glutenfreeoats.com

Oatmega

www.oatmega.com

Snack bars made from natural ingredients.

* Pamela's Products

www.pamelasproducts.com

Cookies, biscotti, and baking mixes.

* The Really Great Food Company

www.reallygreatfood.com

A gluten-free specialty company producing a variety of baking mixes.

* Ronzoni

www.ronzoni.com

A four-grain blend of gluten-free pasta.

Rudi's Gluten-Free Bakery

www.rudisbakery.com/gluten-free

Breads, bars, and wraps.

Schär

www.schar.com

A gluten-free specialty company with a variety of mixes, baked goods, and pastas.

Simple Mills

www.simplemills.com

Gluten-free crackers, cookies, almond flour baking mixes, frosting, and bars.

Snyder's of Hanover
www.snydersofhanover.com
Pretzels.

Tate's Bake Shop
www.tatesbakeshop.com
Cookies and bars.

* Tinkyáda
www.tinkyada.com
A gluten-free specialty company producing an array of rice pastas.

* Udi's
http://udisglutenfree.com
Breads, bagels, muffins, cookies, and granola.

Van's
www.vansfoods.com
Frozen waffles, pancakes, cereals, crackers, snack bars, etc.

* WOW Baking Company
www.wowbaking.com
Baked goods including cookies and mixes.

You can find gluten-free products in almost any supermarket these days, and some chains even have dedicated aisles or sections for gluten-free items. Here's a short list of supermarkets:

City Market	Stop & Shop
Dillons	Trader Joe's
Kroger	Wegmans
Publix	Whole Foods Market

GLOSSARY

Adrenocorticotropic hormone (ACTH): The hormone that stimulates the release of cortisol from the adrenal glands.

Alleles: Different forms of a given gene.

Alopecia areata: An autoimmune disease characterized by hair loss, usually in patches, anywhere on the body.

Amylase: An enzyme secreted by the salivary glands and pancreas that breaks down starches (carbohydrates) into simple sugars.

Anaphylactic shock: A sudden, severe systemic allergic reaction to a substance that causes an IgE-mediated immune response. Symptoms can be mild or potentially life-threatening. It can affect the skin, blood pressure, breathing, and digestion.

Antibody: Antibodies are proteins secreted by cells of the immune system. They are found in the bloodstream and body tissues and protect them from various foreign substances and infections. See *immunoglobulin*.

Antigen: Any foreign material that triggers an immune response.

Antigliadin antibodies (AGA): A food antibody that targets the protein found in wheat.

Antinuclear antibodies (ANA): Antibodies found commonly in autoimmune conditions such as lupus. They also occur in celiac disease and normal people, especially as they age.

Aphthous stomatitis: Canker sores present in the mouth.

Arrythmias: Irregular heartbeats.

Ataxia: A balance disturbance that affects motor control and coordination.

Avascular necrosis: A condition affecting the round bones—the heel, knee, shoulder, hip—where bone cells die because of decreased blood supply. The bone tissue degenerates and becomes "necrotic," i.e., dies. The bone or joint may need to be replaced.

Bacterial overgrowth: A disease characterized by an increase in the number of bacteria in the small intestine by bacteria that normally inhabit the colon. The bacteria cause poor fat and carbohydrate (sugar) absorption. The bacteria also use vitamin B_{12} for their own growth, causing B_{12} deficiency in the body.

Barrett's esophagus: An abnormality of the lining of the lower esophagus due to chronic reflux, considered premalignant.

Bile: A liver secretion that aids in the digestion of fats.

Bile duct: The duct that connects the liver to the small intestine and enables bile to be released into the center of the intestine (lumen).

Bilirubin: The waste product of red blood cells that is excreted by the liver into the intestine.

Bolus: The ball of chewed food formed in the mouth that travels down the esophagus to the stomach.

Bolus of insulin: The extra dose of insulin taken by a diabetic before a meal or snack to control or cover the glucose in the food.

Brush border: The microvilli or tiny "hairs" covering the villi of the small intestine that (1) increase the absorptive area of the small intestine and (2) contain specific enzymes that aid in digestion. When the microvilli are flattened or destroyed, both of these functions are impaired or halted.

Cardiomyopathy: A disease in which the heart muscle becomes inflamed and function is impaired.

CCK (cholecystokinin): A hormone released by the small intestine that has numerous stimulating actions on the pancreas, gallbladder, and intestine. It is an important player in digestion and intestinal motility.

Cerebral calcification: A calcium deposit in the brain.

Chronic pancreatitis: Chronic inflammation of the pancreas resulting in its scarring and atrophy and leading to reduced pancreatic function. It can cause abdominal pain and a malabsorption syndrome.

Chyme: The soupy solution formed in the stomach, consisting of food, gastric juices, enzymes, and saliva.

Clonal lymphocytes: An abnormal proliferation in the number of one type of white blood cell normally seen in malignancies.

Coeliac disease: A spelling of *celiac disease* used outside of the United States.

Colon: The lower end of the digestive tract.

Colostomy: The surgical externalization of the colon to an opening on the belly.

Cortisol: One of the hormones secreted by the adrenal glands.

Crypts: The valleys between the intestinal villi that secrete fluids into the lumen. The main function of the crypts is regenerative, forming and replacing the epithelial cells that layer each villus of the small intestine.

Crypt hyperplasia/hypertrophy: A compensatory mechanism resulting in increased cellular proliferation in the crypts as a result of villous atrophy. The crypts increase their activity in an attempt to replace the villi that are damaged.

Cyclosporins: A class of drugs that affect/alter immune systems in the body. An immunomodulator.

Cytokines: Protein "messengers" produced by inflammatory cells that increase the inflammatory response.

Deamidate: A process involving change in the chemical structure of a compound. Tissue transglutaminase (tTG) deamidates gliadin, changing its molecular structure and enabling it to bind to specific cells, which causes part of the inflammatory response in celiac disease.

Dementia: Disorientation and/or impairment of mental processes caused by disease, old age, trauma, stroke, or unknown factors.

Dermal papillae: A part of the second layer of skin under the top, outer layer.

Dermatitis herpetiformis: An extremely itchy, blistering skin condition that is caused by IgA deposits in the layers of the skin. If you have a definitive diagnosis of dermatitis herpetiformis, you have celiac disease.

Dilated (congestive) cardiomyopathy: The type of cardiomyopathy found in celiac disease in which the heart becomes dilated.

Dipeptides: Proteins are composed of amino acid "chains" held together by peptide bonds. They are split by enzymes (see *peptidases*) into smaller and smaller molecules that can be easily digested. These "chains" come in many different sizes—dipeptides (two amino acids), tripeptides, oligopeptides (*oligo* means "few"), and polypeptides (*poly* means "many").

Duodenum: The upper third of the small intestine.

Dyspepsia: Indigestion/general discomfort in the upper gastrointestinal tract. It may be pain, fullness, or pressure.

Emulsification: The process through which fats are broken into small particles with a surface area that can unite or bind with water in order to pass through the intestinal wall. An emulsifying agent such as phospholipids keeps the droplets from re-forming back into larger drops.

Endocrine glands: A group of glands that help to regulate and synchronize all the other systems of the body by secreting specific hormones. These hormones are the messengers that stimulate and regulate functions throughout the body. The major endocrine glands are the pituitary, pineal, thyroid, parathyroid, adrenal, testes, and ovaries. Endocrine cells are also found in the pancreas, kidneys, liver, thymus, hypothalamus, heart, stomach, and duodenum.

Endopeptidases: Brush border enzymes of the small intestine that break down peptide chains (amino acids) into smaller ones suitable for absorption.

Endoscopy: A minimally invasive procedure during which a small tube with a built-in camera is introduced through the mouth, and advanced through the esophagus, stomach, and upper part of the small intestine. It can help to take pictures or take tissue samples.

Epigenetics: Environmental factors that change the expression of a gene, not the underlying DNA.

Epithelial lymphocytosis: An increased number of lymphocytes within the epithelial cells lining the intestinal mucosa. Seen only under a microscope.

Erythrocyte sedimentation rate (ESR): A blood test to determine levels of inflammation in the body.

Etiology: The origins and causes of a disease.

Exocrine glands: These are glands that secrete fluids through ducts into the lumen (center) of an organ in response to stimuli from the organ. Exocrine glands include the salivary and sweat glands. Other glands such as the pancreas have exocrine cells and endocrine functions.

Ferritin: The storage form of iron in the body.

Fibromyalgia: A condition characterized by fatigue, muscle and joint pain, and GI symptoms. The condition is typically diagnosed when tests cannot match any of these symptoms with another known underlying disease entity or cause.

Fibrosis: The abnormal growth of tissue that eventually scars and blocks an organ.

Gastric acid: The highly effective—and highly corrosive—acid that helps to digest the food in the stomach. It is also protective against infections.

Gastrin: A hormone produced by the stomach that stimulates the release of gastric acid.

Gastroenteritis: Irritation and inflammation of the digestive tract by, e.g., food or pathogens, resulting in gastrointestinal symptoms.

Gastroparesis: Delayed emptying of the stomach. May be caused by decreased intestinal motility due to diabetes, scleroderma, or celiac disease.

Gestational diabetes: A type of diabetes that occurs during pregnancy and usually resolves once the baby is born.

GI: Gastrointestinal.

Gliadin: The alcohol-soluble fraction of gluten found in wheat; the most studied portion in celiac disease, but not necessarily the only toxic fraction in grains.

Gluten: The storage protein of wheat. Essentially, the portion of wheat flour that makes it sticky. The gluten fraction that is most studied in celiac disease is called gliadin, but there are other proteins that chemically resemble gliadin in rye (secalins) and barley (hordeins). These proteins are not strictly glutens, but are generally included in the term and are toxic to people with celiac disease.

Glycosuria: The presence of sugar in the urine, a sign of diabetes.

Hemolytic anemia: A condition characterized by the destruction of red blood cells that results in anemia.

Homeostasis: Essentially, the various forms of balance maintained in the body. In the digestive tract, it is the balance between the secretory and inhibitory mechanisms of digestion; in the nervous system, between the excitory and inhibitory action of neurons.

Hordeins: See *gluten*.

Human leukocyte antigens (HLA): Proteins that sit on the surface of white blood cells and play an important role in the immune system by reacting with foreign substances. These proteins are genetically determined, every person receiving one set from each parent.

Hyperglycemia: High blood glucose levels commonly seen in diabetics who do not have enough, or any, insulin, which is required to metabolize the glucose for use by the body. Usually apparent after a meal.

Hyperthyroidism: Also called thyrotoxicosis. Graves' disease is an autoimmune disease in which the thyroid gland produces too much thyroid hormone, causing the metabolism to speed up. People who are hyperthyroid may have symptoms such as tremors, an increased heart rate and blood pressure, diarrhea, or abnormal menstrual periods.

Hypoglycemia: Low blood glucose levels commonly observed when too much insulin is administered, or too little food eaten to cover the insulin given.

Hypothyroidism: Hypothyroidism is a lack of thyroid hormone. Hashimoto's disease is an autoimmune disease in which the thyroid stops (or decreases) production of hormone and the metabolism slows down. This may affect every body function from digestion to heartbeat.

IgA nephropathy: Also called Berger's disease, IgA nephritis, or IgA glomerulonephritis. An immune disorder that causes IgA (immunoglobulin A) to be deposited in the filters (glomeruli) of the kidney, where they cause inflammation and eventually scarring that impairs kidney function.

Ileitis: An inflammation of the ileum.

Ileostomy: The externalization of the ileum that is opened onto the belly surface.

Ileum: The third segment of the small intestine, or the distal small intestine.

Immunofluorescence: A staining technique that enables labs to isolate and highlight cellular pathology in order to view it under a microscope.

Immunoglobulin A (IgA): The antibodies secreted by plasma cells into the blood or into the lining of the GI tract that act locally in the lining or on the surface to disinfect our ingested food.

Immunoglobulin E (IgE): The antibody that is involved in allergic responses.

Immunoglobulin G (IgG): One of the most numerous antibodies in the body that participates in various immune events.

Inflammatory bowel disease (IBD): Chronic inflammation of the digestive tract of unclear cause. Includes both ulcerative colitis and Crohn's disease.

Insulin-dependent diabetes mellitus (IDDM): Also known as type 1 diabetes or juvenile-onset diabetes; it's characterized by decreased or total absence of insulin.

Interferon: A protein released when the body senses foreign matter, i.e., viruses. It stimulates healthy blood cells to produce substances to fight the infection.

Interferon gamma: A cytokine that is activated by a specific immune response. Interferon gamma enhances the ability of macrophages to kill specific foreign bodies. It is the main cytokine responsible for villous atrophy.

Irritable bowel syndrome (IBS): Any persistent condition with diarrhea and/or constipation, gas, and abdominal pain that is not explained by other known diseases.

Jejunum: The second section of the small intestine.

Ketoacidosis: A toxic buildup of ketones and acids in the bloodstream.

Ketones: A product of fatty acid metabolism. An insulin deficiency causes hyperglycemia, in which glucose is overabundant in the bloodstream but unavailable for use by the cells. The body taps fat and protein for energy, which produces ketones.

Ketosis: A state of continued fat metabolism and ketone release.

Lachrymal glands: The glands surrounding the eyes that supply tears to lubricate the eyeballs.

Lactase: The brush border enzyme of the small intestine that digests milk products.

Lactose intolerance: A condition in which lactase is not produced by the small intestine. Secondary lactose intolerance can occur when the brush border of the small intestine is damaged or destroyed and unable to produce the enzyme.

Lamina propria: Part of the mucosa (lining) of the intestine. The layer of the intestinal wall directly under the epithelial cells covering each villus.

Leukopenia: A condition in which there are not enough white blood cells available in the bloodstream to fight infections.

Linear IgA disease: A rare, blistering disorder that can be mistaken for dermatitis herpetiformis.

Lipase(s): The group of enzymes that break down fats into smaller and smaller components, which are able to be absorbed by the body. It is mainly secreted by the pancreas, but also by salivary glands (lingual lipase).

Lumen: The central, hollow portion of the digestive tube that is the site for the majority of digestive action.

Lupus or systemic lupus erythematosus (SLE): An autoimmune disease in which the immune system attacks the various tissues within the body, leading to organ damage and dysfunction.

Lymphatics: The third part of the vascular system—in addition to veins and arteries—that occurs throughout the body and takes up tissue fluid (lymph). The lymphatics in the villi transport fat to the circulatory system.

Lymphocytes: A type of white blood cell that forms a part of the immune system of the body. Both B and T lymphocytes respond to different antigens in the body.

Macrophages: The Pac-Men of the immune system that engulf and destroy bacteria and microorganisms that enter the bloodstream. They in turn release chemicals that further activate an inflammatory response.

Melanocytes: The cells that make pigment in the skin.

Microscopic colitis: An autoimmune inflammatory condition in the colon often associated with celiac disease. It is characterized by diarrhea but no infection, and can vary in severity. It is diagnosed by biopsy.

Microvilli: The tiny "hairlike" projections lining each epithelial cell on the villi that further increase its absorptive potential and make up the brush border.

Monoamines: Neurotransmitters that regulate mood, e.g., serotonin, dopamine, noradrenaline.

Mucosa: The surface or superficial lining of the wall of the intestine. The mucosa consists of the epithelial (single) cell layer, the lamina propria, and a muscle layer.

Multiple sclerosis (MS): An autoimmune condition of the central nervous system (brain and spinal cord) in which the myelin sheath protecting nerves becomes damaged and eventually lost.

Nephropathy: Damage to the cellular structure of the kidneys that results in impaired function and the inability to clean the blood of waste products.

Nerve conduction studies: Tests for nerve damage in which signals are run through nerve paths to determine if the nerve is functioning properly (i.e., conducting the signal and eliciting an appropriate response).

Neuropathy: A condition caused by the inflammation of nerves, resulting in altered sensation, weakness, or an array of other symptoms.

Neutrophils: White blood cells that release chemicals involved in the inflammatory response.

Oropharyngeal: The mouth and throat.

Osteomalacia: A condition in which the bones become demineralized and soft because of vitamin D and calcium deficiencies.

Osteopenia: A precursor to osteoporosis when bones begin to lose both minerals and density. More calcium is being resorbed than rebuilt into bone mass.

Osteoporosis: A loss of bone density and mineralization, making bones fragile and susceptible to fractures. The skeleton is unable to sustain ordinary stresses and weight.

Pancreatitis: An inflammation of the pancreas that, if chronic, can cause scarring and loss of pancreatic exocrine and endocrine function.

Parathyroid hormone (PTH): The hormone responsible for maintaining normal levels of calcium in the bloodstream. PTH increases the resorption of bone, causing calcium to be released into the bloodstream. It also stimulates the activation of vitamin D, which increases the intestinal absorption of calcium. Primary hyperparathyroidism is the result of inappropriate secretion of PTH, which is frequently due to a benign tumor. Secondary hyperparathyroidism is caused by any disease that continually lowers blood calcium levels and stimulates PTH release.

Parenteral feeding: An intravenous tube inserted through a large vein of the body that delivers nutrients directly into the bloodstream, bypassing the digestive tract.

Paresthesia: Numbness and tingling commonly seen in peripheral neuropathies.

Pathological: Pathology is the study of the origin, nature, and course of a disease.

Pepsin: An enzyme secreted by the stomach that breaks down proteins. See *peptidases*.

Peptidases: A group of enzymes, such as pepsin, that break down proteins into amino acids that can be absorbed by the villi of the small intestine.

Peptide bond: The molecular bond that binds two amino acids.

Peripheral neuropathies: Numbness and/or tingling in the hands and feet because of damaged peripheral nerves.

Peristalsis: The undulating contraction of the wall of the digestive tract that moves food down the digestive tube.

Polycystic ovarian disease: An enlargement and/or thickening of the ovaries that can cause infertility.

Primary biliary cirrhosis: An autoimmune liver disease characterized by scarring of the bile ducts and resulting in cirrhosis (fibrosis and scarring). In PBC, the liver loses the ability to excrete bile salts.

Prophylactic: Preventative; e.g., antibiotics are given to some patients prior to a surgical procedure to prevent potential infection.

Protein-losing enteropathy: A medical condition in which the intestine loses its normal integrity and "weeps" protein and fluid instead of absorbing and holding it.

Proximal intestine: The upper portion of the small intestine that includes the duodenum and the upper jejunum.

Resorption: The process through which calcium is removed from bone and returned to the bloodstream.

Retinopathy: Eye conditions caused by impairment of the vascular supply to the area surrounding the retina.

Rheumatoid arthritis: One of the arthritic conditions in which the synovium, or lining, of the joint becomes inflamed. This results in stiffness, swelling, pain, and, eventually, loss of function of the joints.

Salivary glands: The mucous glands in and around the mouth that supply saliva to aid in swallowing and digestion.

Scleroderma: An autoimmune disease that causes thickening and scarring of connective tissue and muscle. It may involve the intestinal muscles.

Secalins: See *gluten*.

Secondary hyperparathyroidism: See *parathyroid hormone*.

Secretin: A hormone released in the duodenum that stimulates the pancreas to secrete digestive enzymes.

Serologies: Blood tests. All of the molecular components of blood can be measured when serum (blood) is drawn and analyzed. Physicians can request specific panels (tests).

Soluble: Able to dissolve in water. See *emulsification*.

Sphincter: A muscle that acts as a break or valve. The esophageal and pyloric sphincter muscles control the entrance of food into the stomach and its exit into the duodenum, respectively. Spasms and/or malfunctions of these sphincters can be extremely painful and cause digestive problems.

Spruce: A tree.

Sprue: An old term used to describe celiac disease.

Squamous cell cancer: The epithelium consists of cells that cover and line surfaces throughout the body. Malignancies can occur in any epithelium and are named from the one in which they occur. The squamous epithelium consists of multiple layers of cells stacked on one another that protect the body by keeping foreign materials from passing through it. Squamous epithelia cover our skin, mouth, pharynx, and esophagus as well as anus and vagina. This epithelium compares with that lining the digestive tract that consists of a single layer of cells that selectively allow the passage of secretions and nutrients.

Steatorrhea: Fatty, loose stools because of the presence of increased fat in them.

Substrate: The medium to which blood and cells are added for lab analysis. It may consist of human or animal tissue or fluids and enables the lab to activate or freeze the test material for observation.

Sucrase: An enzyme that breaks down sugars into glucose.

Tenesmus: The feeling of incomplete evacuation. A common symptom in acute diarrhea, colitis, and irritable bowel syndrome.

Thyroiditis: An inflammation/disease process of the thyroid gland.

Tissue transglutaminase (tTG): tTG is a family of enzymes that is found in every tissue of the body and joins proteins together. It reacts with gliadin, setting off the chain of reactions that destroys the villi of the small intestine in celiac disease.

Triglycerides: Dietary fats that must be broken down in the small intestine into glycerol and fatty acids in order to be absorbed by the mucosa. They are insoluble in water until they are broken into these smaller components.

Trypsin: An enzyme secreted by the pancreas that breaks down protein.

tTG: See *tissue transglutaminase.*

Tumor necrosis factor: A cytokine that stimulates inflammation.

Type 1 diabetes (IDDM): See *insulin-dependent diabetes mellitus.*

Villi: Small projections lining the wall of the small intestine that greatly increase its absorptive power; lined with epithelial cells covered in microvilli that absorb nutrients.

Villous atrophy: The inflammation and eventual flattening (loss) of the villi of the small intestine, resulting in a decreased surface for absorption.

Vitiligo: Vitiligo (vit-ill-EYE-go) is a loss of pigmentation of the skin in which white patches of skin appear on different parts of the body.

INDEX

Page references in *italics* indicate figures.

About the Authors

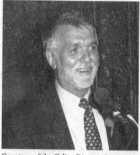

Courtesy of the Celiac Disease Center at
Columbia University

PETER H. R. GREEN, M.D., is the director of the Celiac Disease Center at Columbia University. He is the Phyllis and Ivan Seidenberg Professor of Medicine at the College of Physicians and Surgeons, Columbia University, and attending physician at the Columbia University Medical Center (New York-Presbyterian Hospital). Celiac disease has been his focus for more than thirty years with equal concentration on patient care and research. He is also the coauthor of *Gluten Exposed: The Science Behind the Hype and How to Navigate to a Healthy, Symptom-Free Life.*

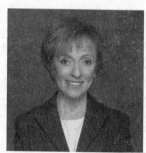

by AnnieWatson.com

RORY JONES, M.S., is a medical writer and adjunct professor of narrative medicine at Barnard College of Columbia University. She has done extensive work on health and medical topics, including educational programs for both adults and children. She specializes in "translating" scientific information for a consumer audience. Diagnosed with celiac disease in 1998, she has researched and written about it and the gluten-free diet for medical as well as consumer publications. She is also the coauthor of *Gluten Exposed: The Science Behind the Hype and How to Navigate to a Healthy, Symptom-Free Life.*

ALSO BY DR. PETER H.R. GREEN AND RORY JONES, M.S.

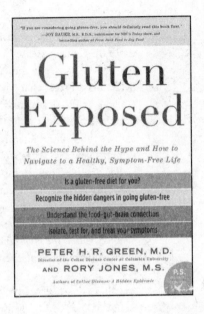

The one book you should read if you are on a gluten-free diet or plan to go gluten-free.

"There's a lot of confusion surrounding gluten—whether eliminating it can help you lose weight, clear brain fog, cure stomach issues and more. The brilliant and renowned Dr. Peter Green, and science writer Rory Jones, have cut through the confusion to provide evidence-based answers and advice you can trust. . . . They sort through all the science to create a comprehensive guide on the subject. If you are considering going gluten-free, you should definitely read this book first."

— Joy Bauer, MS, RDN, nutritionist for NBC's TODAY show, founder of Nourish Snacks
and best-selling author of *From Junk Food to Joy Food*